A Profile of
Health and Disease
in America

Diabetes, Liver, and Digestive Disease

Wrynn Smith, Ph.D.

Facts On File Publications
New York, New York   •   Oxford, England

**A Profile of Health and Disease in America:
Diabetes, Liver, and Digestive Disease**

copyright © 1988 by Wrynn Smith

Library of Congress Cataloging-in-Publication Data
Smith, Wrynn.
    Diabetes, liver, and digestive disease.

    (A Profile of health and disease in America)
    Bibliography: p.
    Includes index.
    1. Digestive organs—Diseases—United States—
Statistics.   2. Liver—Diseases—United States—Statistics.   3. Diabetes—United States—Statistics.
4. Kidneys—Diseases—United States—Statistics.
I. Title. II. Series: Smith, Wrynn. Profile of Health
and Disease in America. [DNLM: 1. Diabetes Mellitus—
occurrence—United States.   2. Digestive System
Diseases—occurrence—United States.   3. Kidney Diseases—
occurrence—United States.   4. Liver Diseases—
occurrence—United States. WI 100 S664d]
RA645.D54S65 1988   614.5′9462′00973021   87-24532
ISBN 0-8160-1459-0
ISBN 0-8160-1588-0 (7 volume set)

Series design: Jo Stein

British CIP data available on request

Printed in the United States of America

10 9 8 7 6 5 4 3 2 1

Contents

Preface

Just a few decades ago, treating the sick was a simple affair. The local family doctor, equipped with a small array of poultices and a sympathetic manner, did his best to fight disease. Knowledge, medicines, instrumentation, and surgical procedures developed slowly. Today, however, in the era of proliferating biotechnology, specialization, third-party financing, hospices, and surgicenters, medical school professors seem to relish telling their students that 50% of what they are learning will be obsolete five years after graduation.

The flow of information crossing the desk of busy health-care professionals trying to keep abreast of ever-accelerating developments in disease diagnosis, treatment, and prevention, as well as in the financing, organization, and delivery of health care, is often overwhelming. Clearly, the need to keep up is critical. To be informed, health-care professionals—be they practitioners, hospital administrators, health-care planners, policy makers, insurers, or hospital or pharmaceutical supply executives—must attend to material from many disconnected sources. These sources might include current editions of classic texts, weekly and monthly professional journals, current research papers presented at colloquia, and a steady stream of government bulletins and study publications from the Centers for Disease Control, NIH, the Center for Health Statistics, and foundation reports. As with the proverbial forest that can't be seen for the trees, the voluminous and fragmented form of this information often obscures the major changes and trends rapidly occurring in the health care field.

The task of a grant applicant to locate and collate statistical information when framing the need for his work is a research project in itself. The same is true of a researcher defining a hypothesis, a physician determining the current utilization of a particular therapy regimen or a hospital administrator projecting bed needs.

To help such workers and investigators, I decided to gather data from many sources into one comprehensive coordinated source, this series entitled *A Profile of Health and Disease in America,* that will serve as a handy and definitive resource tool for health professionals.

Each volume contains both historical and current statistics on the incidence, prevalence, and mortality of major diseases within one of the major medical specialties. I've presented data for different geographic areas within the United States as well as international data. I've also included information on the use of various medicines and surgical procedures. The length of a hospital stay, how it varies geographically or for patients based on sex, and treatment costs are included as are discussions of major controversies. Thus, the reader will easily find data on flu viruses, changes in virus strains, current fertility rates of American teenagers, changes in the obesity level of Americans, and the latest incidence of pertussis, with a discussion of the pros and cons of the pertussis vaccine and of how many men suffer from toxic shock syndrome. Those readers interested in digestive disease can find recent information from government surveys on problems as diverse as ulcers and hemorrhoids. The volume on mental disease provides a wealth of data on depressive symptomatology, drug usage, alcoholism, and homicide and puts the recent increase of teenage suicide in historical perspective.

Data sources include the 1983 Symposium on Cancer Treatment; Public Health Reports; the National Natality Survey; the NHANES Surveys; publications of the Atlanta Centers for Disease Control; and NIH publications, as well as those of the American Heart, Lung, and Blood Institute, The American Cancer Institute, and the Institute for Allergy and Infectious Disease. Published research articles are discussed and referenced, and each volume includes a bibliography that can be used by those seeking to go beyond initial review of pertinent health data. These comprehensive volumes on so many health topics need not be the last source consulted, but I think for those owning them they will always be the first.

Introduction

Digestive diseases elicit less attention and fewer headlines than do cancer and cardiovascular diseases. Yet health expenditures for digestive diseases in the United States ranked second highest after cardiovascular disease in 1981 at $32 billion compared to $33 billion for the latter.

Adults younger than age 65 years suffer more from digestive diseases than from any other kind. More than one half of them suffer from some digestive disease, including 20 million who have a chronic digestive disability. An estimated 100 million experience intermittent bouts of digestive disease. In 1980, 75,202 deaths were attributable to digestive diseases. This statistic accounted for 3.8% of the overall mortality for that year. This did not include deaths from diabetes or renal disease (also discussed in this volume).

Much of the prevalence data in this volume was gathered from the National Digestive Diseases Advisory Board Report, 1983; the National Health Interview Surveys of 1968, 1975, and 1981; the National Ambulatory Medical Care Survey, 1981; the National Hospital Discharge Survey, 1980; and several other federal government publications. As with other volumes in this series, data from past surveys facilitate the detection of trends and comparison of environmental variables that may be contributing factors to disease. Despite a precipitous decline in some digestive diseases—such as ulcers and more recently alcohol-related cirrhosis—digestive diseases are becoming more prevalent. Contrary to popular belief, women develop hernias and esophageal bleeding almost as often as men. More in keeping with expectation, women do suffer from constipation and gallbladder disorders more than men. Interestingly, there is a consistent association between digestive-disease prevalence and lower socioeconomic status. The prevalence of both ulcers and liver disease increases as one goes from east to west in the United States.

Liver disease accounts for more morbidity and bed-days than any other digestive disease, excluding diabetes and renal disease. Forty years ago, nothing was known about one of the leading causes of liver disease—hepatitis B. But progress since the 1969 discovery of the Au antigen associated with hepatitis B has been noteworthy. Scientists at the National Institutes of Health (NIH) estimate that the antigen screening test to detect hepatitis B in blood banks saves the United States $500 million annually in health-care costs. The potential of more recently developed vaccines for the hepatitis-B and A viruses to relieve the burden of hepatic morbidity and mortality is even more impressive when one realizes that an estimated 200 million people worldwide are chronically infected with hepatitis B.

The rate of hepatitis B in the United States is 24.1 per 100,000, surpassing the hepatitis-A rate for the first time in 1983, although both forms are thought to be greatly under-reported. Detailed data about the prevalence of the three major forms of hepatitis in each state, and for people by age, sex, racial background, and occupation are presented in Chapter 3, together with a discussion of the connections between hepatitis B, cirrhosis, and liver cancer.

The upward trend of cirrhosis began reversing itself in 1973. By 1984 incidence fell from 15.9 per 100,000 to 11.4. Before this downward trend, the rate for black males had increased from 12.6 per 100,000 in 1960 to 26.7 in 1973. White males also showed an increase from 15.6 to 20.5 as of 1973. Alcohol-related cirrhosis deaths between 1968 and 1977 totaled 121,256. The reversal and current trend in cirrhosis mortality may be attributable to advances in controlling hepatitis, the advent of liver transplant technology, and changes in the pattern of alcohol consumption.

The estimated prevalence of diabetes, another major disease related to digestion and metabolism, is 12 million as of 1985. Reflections on interpreting the glucose tolerance test (Chapter 4) underscore the difficulty of detecting diabetes early and current under estimates of prevalence and mortality. In 1984, 35,804 deaths were directly attributable to diabetes. But the many life-threatening complications of the disease such as renal failure and cardiovascular disease suggest that the true mortality attributable to diabetes as the primary cause of death is much greater than reported.

The general consensus based on many studies of diverse diabetic populations is that the disease shortens the normal lifespan by one-third. The death rate in juvenile-onset diabetes patients is 11 times higher than it is in the nondiabetic population. In addition to mortality, epidemiologic studies have identified several risk factors associated with the development of diabetes, including genetic ones and obesity.

Studies reviewed by the Diabetes Data Group in 1977 of various American cities show that cardiovascular and renal complications were the preeminent causes of death in long-term, Type II diabetics. Other studies indicate that gangrene and amputation are 20 times more likely to occur in diabetics than in nondiabetics, whereas ketoacidosis accounts for 10% of deaths among diabetics.

Approximately 9.5 million office visits were related primarily or secondarily to diabetes. Exogenous insulin accounted for 18% of all drug mentions during these visits. In 1981, the cost of this and other types of care totaled $7.9 billion.

Renal diseases (ICDA 580-589) classified as nephritis, nephrotic syndrome, and nephrosis constitute the 15th leading cause of death in the United States. In 1983, fatalities totaled 18,710. Since 1950, the death rate has been declining (falling from 17 to 8 per 100,000). But as the End Stage Renal Disease Program data indicate, the number of participants with serious renal disease in the federal government's Medicare program has risen from 18,410 in 1974 to 70,055 in 1982. Those patients requiring dialysis were treated in 1,218 facilities (689 hospitals and 529 independent facilities).

Increasing costs underscore efforts to train patients in self-assisted and home dialysis techniques, including continuous ambulatory peritoneal dialysis. Indeed, the percentage of patients receiving home dialysis has risen from 13% in 1979 to almost 17.8% in 1982.

The mortality rate of dialysis patients is highest for white males (142 per 1,000); many such patients are awaiting a kidney transplant. Graft retention rates for cadaver vs. living, related-donor transplants are compared in Chapter 5, as are the costs and charges of the two types of donated kidney reported for various cities.

The proportion of patients receiving a transplant compared to those waiting for a kidney has declined in recent years. The charges for hospital stays for those receiving dialysis and those who have received a transplant are also compared for patients by age as are the mortality rates for the two forms of treatment. The longest survivors following complete renal failure are those who received a kidney from a sibling. Yet the costs in securing an organ and of hospitalization associated with transplants, including rejection episodes, make this option possible for only a limited portion of the patients on dialysis. Continuing advances will, it is hoped, eventually make both transplants and dialysis technology more effective and lasting—as well as less expensive—solutions to kidney failure than either one is today.

The Problem Of Digestive Diseases 1

Cardiovascular and circulatory diseases account for the greatest annual expenditure of health-care resources in the United States. But digestive-disease costs run a close second. In 1980, when circulatory diseases cost the nation $33 billion, digestive diseases cost $32 billion, including $15 billion spent on dental care. This did not include expenditure for metabolic diseases, such as diabetes or hepatic disease. Digestive diseases absorbed 61% of professional-service expenditures, 15% of nursing-home expenditures, and 13% of all drug expense.

Medical costs for digestive disorders were highest among all diseases for adults younger than age 65 years. They accounted for 18% of medical monies paid out by both men and women. Digestive diseases were also among the five most costly categories of disease for those older than age 65 years. In 1980, per capita expenditure for those older than age 65 years suffering from digestive diseases was $213 for men and $223 for women. Those younger than age 65 years in 1980 spent $110 if male and $143 if female. Digestive diseases ranked first in per capita expenditure in the young patient and third in the old patient.

Digestive diseases may be classified as either acute or chronic. The division is arbitrary at best because someone may experience a single, acute gallbladder attack for which he is hospitalized and undergoes surgery or he can suffer acute gallbladder attacks chronically over many years. Someone may have a limited bout of ulcers requiring hospitalization or medical treatment after which the ulcer heels and he has no further problem. He may, on the other hand, suffer chronically from ulcers. In many instances acute attacks occur within a long-standing pattern of chronic disease. Hence, the emphasis in digestive-disease data collection is primarily for chronic illness.

In 1980, nonmalignant digestive diseases were the causes of death for 75,202 persons in the United States, accounting for 3.8% of annual total mortality. Digestive diseases do not arouse much concern because they are not regarded as life threatening in the way that cancer or heart disease is. Yet, digestive diseases, which are often fatal, also contribute to much of the illness people experience daily. Indeed, more than one-half of the U.S. population currently suffers from digestive disease (excluding diabetes or renal disease).

Surveys of otherwise healthy American adults indicate that about one out of four has more than six episodes of abdominal pain in a given year, whereas 17% reported symptoms of bowel dysfunction. An estimated 20 million Americans suffer chronic forms of digestive disease; another 14 million suffer acute episodes, and 100 million suffer intermittent bouts of digestive disease. These reports represent 8% who have chronic disease problems, 43% with intermittent pain and 6% who suffer acute attacks (Fig. 1–1.) These percentages will undoubtedly rise as the population ages and more people develop these chronic and debilitating disorders.

FIG. 1–1.   U.S. population affected by digestive diseases

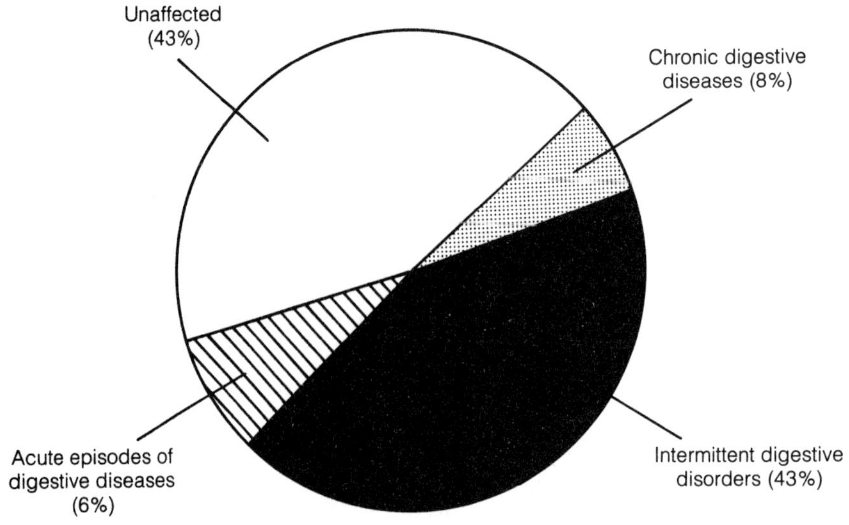

Unaffected (43%)
Chronic digestive diseases (8%)
Acute episodes of digestive diseases (6%)
Intermittent digestive disorders (43%)

Source: *National Digestive Diseases Advisory Board Report*, 1983

INCIDENCE AND PREVALENCE

The prevalence of several major digestive diseases in 1980 by sex and age is shown in Table 1–1.

The data in Table 1–1 are similar to those collected in 1975 when another complete federal survey was done on the prevalence and incidence of these diseases. The overall prevalence of the 9 most widespread digestive diseases listed in Table 1–1 totals about 23 million as reported for the noninstitutionalized civilian population. This is 1 million more than the number reported in 1975. This rise occurred despite a fall during the last decade in the incidence of several digestive diseases, such as stomach ulcers. The prevalence of 11 selected digestive diseases and their rate per 1,000 of population in 1975 is shown in Table 1–2. The reported ulcer and gallbladder conditions listed in Table 1–1 are fewer than those reported in Table 1–2.

TABLE 1–1. Persons with Nine Selected Reported Chronic Digestive Conditions: Rates per 1,000 Persons by Sex, Age, and Conditions, United States, 1980

| | | SEX | | | AGE | | | |
| | | | | | RATE | | | |
CONDITION	NUMBER PER 1,000	Both sexes, all ages	Male	Female	Under 17	17–44	45–64	65+
Ulcer of stomach/ duodenum	3,615	16.6	16.5	16.6	0.4*	17.7	30.4	26.2
Frequent constipation	3,579	16.4	7.6	24.6	6.1	11.4	20.5	53.6
Hernia of abdominal cavity	3,888	17.8	19.1	16.7	3.2*	7.7	37.6	56.4
Functional and symptomatic upper gastrointestinal disorder	3,720	17.1	19.5	14.8	1.9*	16.3	27.2	38.1
Gallbladder condition	1,217	5.6	2.9	8.1	—*	3.6	10.7	17.3
Gastritis and duodenitis	1,706	7.8	6.9	8.7	1.3*	7.4	13.3	15.2
Diverticula of intestine	1,380	6.3	2.7	9.7	—*	0.6*	14.9	28.3
Chronic enteritis/ colitis	2,293	10.5	7.0	13.8	4.3	9.3	15.0	22.1
Intestinal condition	1,649	7.6	4.2	10.7	0.4*	5.8	18.4	12.0

*Does not meet standards of reliability
Source: *National Digestive Diseases Advisory Board Report*, 1983

TABLE 1–2.   Number and Rate per 1,000 Persons, of Selected Chronic Digestive Conditions Reported in Health Interviews: United States, 1975

CHRONIC CONDITION AND ICDA CODE*		CONDITIONS IN THOUSANDS	RATE PER 1,000 PERSONS
Ulcer of stomach and duodenum	531–534	3,955	18.9
Frequent constipation	564.0	3,811	18.2
Hernia of abdominal cavity	550–553	3,725	17.8
Functional and symptomatic upper gastrointestinal disorder†	536, 784.0, 784.1, 784.3, 784.7, 785.4 pt.	3,462	16.6
Gallbladder condition‡	574, 575, 576.0, 576.1, 576.9	1,625	7.8
Gastritis and duodenitis	535	1,465	7.0
Diverticula of intestine	562	1,323	6.3
Chronic enteritis and ulcerative colitis	563	1,183	5.7
Intestinal condition**	564.1, 564.9, 785.4 pt.	876	4.2
Stomach trouble, N.O.S.		501	2.4
Liver condition¶	570–573	411	2.0

*Eighth Revision International Classification of Diseases, Adapted for Use in the United States, 1965
†Gas (pains) in stomach were coded to ICDA coce 536; in intestines, to ICDA code 564
‡Includes gallbladder trouble N.O.S.
**Includes intestinal or bowel trouble N.O.S.
¶Includes hepatitis or liver trouble N.O.S.
Note: N.O.S. = not otherwise specified
Source: Vital and Health Statistics, Series 10, No. 115

TABLE 1–3. Prevalence and Incidence of Selected Chronic Digestive Conditions Reported in Health Interviews per 1,000 Persons,* by Age: United States, 1968 and 1975

CHRONIC CONDITION	PREVALENCE PER 1,000 PERSONS								INCIDENCE PER 1,000 PERSONS							
	All Ages		Under 45 years		45–64 years		65 years and over		All ages		Under 45 years		45–64 years		65 years and over	
	1968	1975	1968	1975	1968	1975	1968	1975	1968	1975	1968	1975	1968	1975	1968	1975
Ulcer of stomach and duodenum	17.2	18.9	10.8	12.8	33.4	33.7	29.0	30.8	3.0†	2.9	2.4	2.5	4.1	4.1	4.5	3.5
Frequent constipation	23.8	18.2	10.7	9.4	35.0	23.6	96.3	67.1	2.0	1.6	1.6	1.5	1.8	1.2	5.8	3.3
Hernia of abdominal cavity	16.3	17.8	7.0	6.4	28.3	34.3	58.8	62.2	3.2	3.6	2.1	2.2	4.7	6.0	7.4	8.5
Functional and symptomatic upper gastrointestinal disorder	13.1	16.6	6.7	9.5	23.5	29.4	37.7	38.5	1.6	2.1	1.2	1.8	2.7	3.2	2.5	2.4
Gallbladder condition	10.3	7.8	4.0	3.4	21.4	15.3	32.8	22.0	1.8	1.7	1.0	1.2	3.4	2.9	4.3	3.4
Gastritis and duodenitis	8.6	7.0	4.4	4.2	16.2	11.4	24.0	17.4	1.4	1.5	1.2	1.3	1.8	1.8	2.4	2.2
Diverticula of intestine	...	6.3	...	0.6	...	13.2	...	31.0	...	0.7	...	0.1	...	1.5	...	2.6
Chronic enteritis and ulcerative colitis (excluding diverticula of intestine)	...	5.7	...	3.3	...	9.7	...	13.5	...	0.9	...	0.7	...	1.3	...	1.4
Chronic enteritis and ulcerative colitis (including diverticula of intestine)	9.3	11.1	3.5	3.9	17.9	21.3	34.0	39.2	1.4	0.6	0.7	0.4	2.5	1.2	4.6	0.8†
Intestinal condition	4.2	4.2	1.9	2.5	8.1	6.7	12.5	10.7	0.6	0.6	0.4	0.5	0.9	0.6	1.1	1.0
Stomach trouble, N.O.S.	2.7	2.4	1.6	1.8	5.2	3.1	5.3	5.1	0.4	0.5	0.4	0.5	0.5	0.4	0.6	0.5
Liver condition	1.4	2.0	0.5	1.0	2.4	4.4	5.2	3.7	0.2	0.5	0.2	0.4	0.3	0.7	0.3	0.6

*Number of persons (in thousands) used in computing rates were as follows:

	1968	1975
All ages	195,889	209,065
Under 45 years	137,165	144,683
45–64 years	40,298	43,094
65 years and over	18,426	21,287

†May be unreliable estimate
Note: N.O.S. = not otherwise specified.
Source: Vital and Health Statistics, Series 10, No. 115

TABLE 1–4.   Number and Rate per 1,000 Persons of Selected Chronic Digestive Conditions Reported in Health Interviews by Age and Sex: United States, 1975 (data are based on household interviews of the civilian noninstitutionalized population)

SEX AND SELECTED CHRONIC DIGESTIVE CONDITION	ALL AGES	UNDER 45 YEARS			45–64 YEARS	65 YEARS AND OVER	ALL AGES	UNDER 45 YEARS			45–64 YEARS	65 YEARS AND OVER
		Total	Under 17 years	17–44 years				Total	Under 17 years	17–44 years		
		Number of conditions in thousands						Rate per 1,000 population				
Both sexes												
Ulcer of stomach and duodenum	3,955	1,846	73	1,773	1,453	656	18.9	12.8	1.2	21.4	33.7	30.8
Frequent constipation	3,811	1,367	318	1,049	1,015	1,429	18.2	9.4	5.1	12.7	23.6	67.1
Hernia of abdominal cavity	3,725	924	214	710	1,477	1,324	17.8	6.4	3.5	8.6	34.3	62.2
Functional and symptomatic upper gastrointestinal disorder	3,462	1,373	77	1,296	1,269	820	16.6	9.5	0.2*	15.7	15.3	22.0
Gallbladder condition	1,625	498	14	484	659	469	7.8	3.4	0.2*	5.8	15.3	20.4
Gastritis and duodenitis	1,465	604	71	533	491	370	7.0	4.2	1.1	6.4	11.4	17.4
Diverticula of intestine	1,323	94		94	569	660	6.3	0.6		1.1	13.2	31.0
Chronic enteritis and ulcerative colitis	1,183	479	46	433	416	287	5.7	3.3	0.7	5.2	9.7	13.5
Intestinal condition	876	360	42	318	289	227	4.2	2.5	0.7	3.8	6.7	10.7
Stomach trouble, N.O.S.	501	260	46	214	132	109	2.4	1.8	0.7	2.6	3.1	5.1
Liver condition	411	142	20*	122	189	79	2.0	1.0	0.3*	1.5	4.4	3.7

Male

Ulcer of stomach and duodenum	2,091	962	42	920	805	324	20.7	13.4	1.3	23.0	39.2	36.9
Frequent constipation	902	298	132	166	221	383	8.9	4.2	4.2	4.2	10.8	43.6
Hernia of abdominal cavity	1,954	545	136	409	784	625	19.4	7.6	4.3	10.2	38.2	71.2
Functional and symptomatic upper gastrointestinal disorder	1,747	765	37	729	654	328	17.3	10.7	1.2	18.2	31.8	37.4
Gallbladder condition	304	74	2*	72	137	93	3.0	1.0	0.1*	1.8	6.7	10.6
Gastritis and duodenitis	588	272	36	236	181	135	5.8	3.8	1.1	5.9	8.8	15.4
Diverticula of intestine	366	23*		23	190	153	3.6	0.3*		0.6	9.3	17.4
Chronic enteritis and ulcerative colitis	361	149	27*	122	137	75	3.6	2.1	0.9*	3.1	6.7	8.5
Intestinal condition	246	103	17*	85	82	61	2.4	1.4	0.5*	2.1	4.0	6.9
Stomach trouble, N.O.S.	233	118	22*	96	64	51	2.3	1.6	0.7*	2.4	3.1	5.8
Liver condition	231	74	9*	65	117	40	2.3	1.0	0.3*	1.6	5.7	4.6

Female

Ulcer of stomach and duodenum	1,863	885	31*	853	647	331	17.2	12.1	1.0*	19.9	28.7	26.5
Frequent constipation	2,909	1,069	186	883	793	1,046	26.9	14.6	6.1	20.6	35.2	83.6
Hernia of abdominal cavity	1,771	378	77	301	693	699	16.4	5.2	2.5	7.0	30.7	55.9
Functional and symptomatic upper gastrointestinal disorder	1,715	608	40	568	615	492	15.9	8.3	1.3	13.3	27.3	39.3
Gallbladder condition	1,322	424	12*	411	522	376	12.2	5.8	0.4*	9.6	23.1	30.1
Gastritis and duodenitis	878	332	35	297	311	235	8.1	4.5	1.2	6.9	13.8	18.8
Diverticula of intestine	957	71		71	379	507	8.8	1.0		1.7	16.8	40.5
Chronic enteritis and ulcerative colitis	822	331	20*	311	279	212	7.6	4.5	0.7*	7.3	12.4	17.0
Intestinal condition	631	258	25*	233	206	167	5.8	3.5	0.8*	5.4	9.1	13.4
Stomach trouble, N.O.S.	268	141	24*	118	69	58	2.5	1.9	0.8*	2.8	3.1	4.6
Liver condition	179	68	12*	56	72	40	1.7	0.9	0.4*	1.3	3.2	3.2

*May be unreliable
Source: *Vital and Health Statistics*, Series 10, No. 115

The decreasing incidence of some diseases is evident again when 1975 prevalence data are compared with those gathered seven years earlier (Table 1–3). Although the two surveys had different sampling errors, which make comparison tenuous, overall difference trends likely reflect true differences.

Gallbladder conditions were less common in 1975 than in 1968. The same is true for gastritis and duodenitis. The rate of reported gallbladder conditions decreased from 10.3 per 1,000 to 7.8, a drop of 24%, whereas gastritis and duodenitis decreased by 19%. Conversely, a 27% increase in the prevalence rate of functional and symptomatic upper gastrointestinal disorders between the two survey periods was reported. This occurred even though several diseases included in this group under the Seventh ICDA code were shifted to other disease categories by the Eighth Revision during this period. These changes in prevalence and incidence between 1968 and 1975 in persons of different ages are shown in Table 1–3.

Table 1–4 shows the number and rate of selected digestive diseases for the civilian population by age and sex for 1975. These data portray some interesting and unexpected facts that are even more pronounced in the 1980 data (Table 1–1).

Abdominal hernias are thought to be primarily a male affliction. But the data show that almost as many women have hernias as men. Also, upper gastrointestinal disorders, including those related to drinking, such as bleeding esophagus, are almost as common in women as they are in men. Finally, women who generally eat less and may be less active than men have a much greater problem with constipation and smooth functioning of the intestinal tract than have men. Women also have more gallbladder problems although they probably consume less fat than do men.

Comparison of the differences by age and sex may be easier to discern by looking at their graphic illustration (Figs. 1–2 and 1–3). As Figure 1–2 shows, all of the diseases except ulcers and liver conditions become increasingly common with age. Ulcers and liver conditions show a slightly lower prevalence rate after age 65 years than during age 45 to 64 years. With the exception of ulcers, hernia, liver, and upper gastrointestinal disorders, women have more digestive diseases than men. But the rate of prevalence is typically not large. Gallbladder disease and constipation are two disorders that women seem to experience substantially more than men at 25.9 per 1,000 vs. 8.9 for the latter and 12.2 vs. 3.0 for the former (Fig. 1–3).

The prevalence of these disorders in subjects of different races is shown in Figure 1–4. The data indicate that constipation and upper gastrointestinal difficulties are more common among black and

FIG. 1–2.   Prevalence of selected chronic digestive conditions by age, 1975.

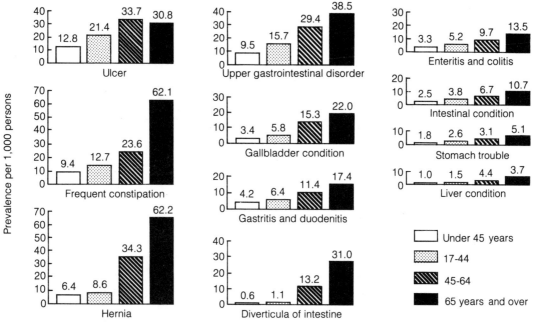

Source: *Vital and Health Statistics,* Series 10, No. 115

FIG. 1–3.   Prevalence of selected chronic digestive conditions by sex, 1975

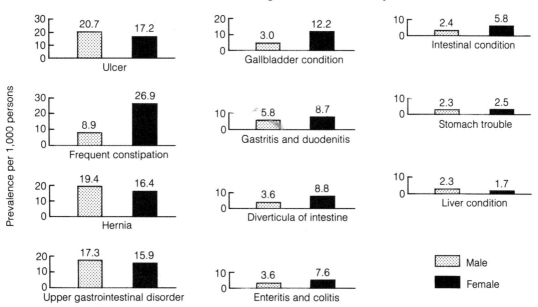

Source: *Vital and Health Statistics,* Series 10, No. 115

FIG. 1–4. Prevalence of selected chronic digestive conditions by race, 1975

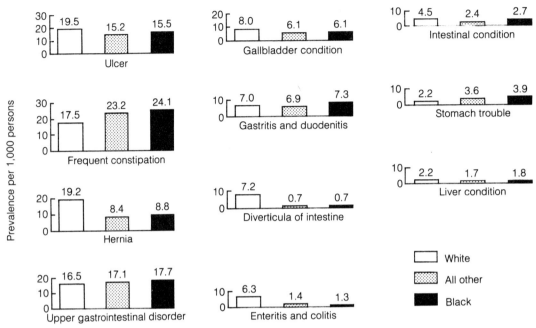

Source: *Vital and Health Statistics*, Series 10, No. 115

other non-whites. But ulcers, hernias, gallbladder disorders, and several intestinal conditions are more common among whites.

Figure 1–5 shows the prevalence of digestive diseases, given one's socioeconomic status. The association with low income is striking for all 11 diseases. The data pose some suggestive questions about the diet of low-income persons, which is known to differ significantly from that of people of higher income.

Figure 1–6 shows the prevalence of the most widespread digestive diseases for different regions of the United States. Although regional variability for different diseases exists, ulcer seems to take a greater toll as one goes from east to west as do liver conditions. Each condition may reflect an east-west pattern of alcohol consumption, which contributes to the two diseases. The South has a higher prevalence of constipation, hernia, upper gastrointestinal disorders, and intestinal, stomach and liver conditions than has any other region of the United States. Because the South also has a higher concentration of poor people than other regions, the prevalence may simply reflect this population. Poor people understandably may be under more stress, and digestive conditions may be triggered by stress. However, the reason may be much more tangi-

FIG. 1–5. Prevalence of selected chronic digestive conditions by family income, 1975

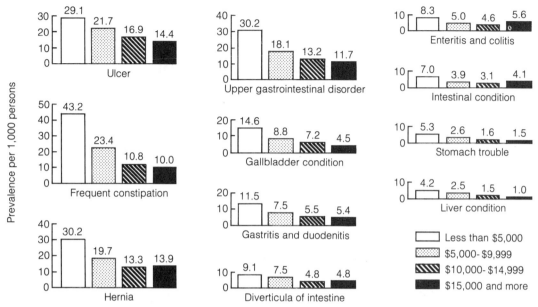

Source: *Vital and Health Statistics,* Series 10, No. 115

FIG. 1-6. Prevalence of selected chronic digestive conditions by region, 1975

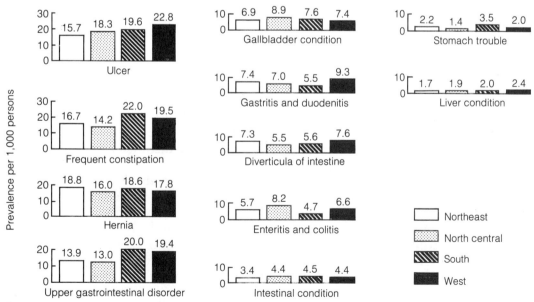

Source: *Vital and Health Statistics,* Series 10, No. 115

ble, such as the dietary habits of Southerners who happen to be poor or the dietary habits of poor people who happen to live more often in the South than elsewhere.

The impact of diet has been established for many diseases. It seems reasonable that diet should certainly have an impact on digestive diseases preeminently. Historically the traditional foods of the American South have been low in protein and quite high in fiber and carbohydrates in the form of peas, beans, and other legumes and leafy vegetables. It is widely recognized that vegetables like cabbage, onions, and beans are difficult to digest and cause flatulence and esophageal regurgitation. This observation is interesting in light of recent recommendations that Americans adopt a high-fiber, high-carbohydrate diet instead of their present high protein, high-fat, high-sugar diet. Nutrition authorities recommend increasing fiber intake gradually (from the current average of 10-15 grams daily to the recommended 30-37 grams) in order to minimize digestive distress. No one recommends a daily fiber intake in excess of 37g, which is known to irritate the intestinal tract.

The Southern diet also appears to be high in fat; many foods, including chicken and potatoes, are deep-fried. It is high in sodium as well. The latter two aspects, rather than fiber intake, may account for some of the digestive disturbances that are more serious than the regurgitation and flatulence provoked by legumes and vegetables.

DISABILITY

The percentage of survey respondents interviewed in 1975 who reported disability because of a digestive or liver disorder in terms of bed-days spent in the year before the interview varied considerably (Table 1–5). Constipation required few days in bed, but 10.7% of those with liver complaints spent 31 or more days in bed. Gallbladder and stomach conditions were responsible for 1 to 3 bed-days in 9.6% of those with the former disorder and in 12.9% of those with the latter.

Episodes requiring treatment by a physician are particularly high for those with liver conditions (Table 1–6). Indeed, 31% reported seeing a physician about their ailment five or more times in the year before the interview. Gallbladder and nonspecific stomach trouble also accounted for several physician visits.

Digestive disease patients with gallbladder and liver conditions, ulcers, and hernias are hospitalized the most, and large numbers of people with various digestive diseases were under doctor-prescribed medication before the survey (Table 1–7).

TABLE 1–5. Selected Chronic Digestive Conditions Reported in Health Interviews and Percentage Distribution of Conditions by Bed-days in the Year Prior to Interview: United States, 1975

| CHRONIC CONDITION | NUMBER OF CONDITIONS (IN THOUSANDS) | NUMBER OF BED-DAYS | | | | | | |
		Total	None	1–3	4–7	8–14	15–30	≥31
		Percent distribution						
Ulcer of stomach and duodenum	3,955	100.0	74.5	7.4	5.2	4.4	3.6	2.2
Frequent constipation	3,811	100.0	94.2	1.9	1.8	0.7*	0.2*	0.3*
Hernia of abdominal cavity	3,725	100.0	75.8	6.2	6.5	4.7	3.0	1.5
Functional and symptomatic upper gastrointestinal disorder	3,462	100.0	89.8	4.3	1.4	1.0*	0.7*	0.6*
Gallbladder condition	1,625	100.0	59.7	9.6	7.0	9.5	7.8	3.5
Gastritis and duodenitis	1,465	100.0	76.8	8.0	6.1	4.1	2.0	1.2*
Diverticula of intestine	1,323	100.0	81.5	4.1	5.1	3.9	2.3*	1.3*
Chronic enteritis and ulcerative colitis	1,183	100.0	76.1	6.9	6.2	4.1	2.0*	1.9*
Intestinal condition	876	100.0	82.0	6.4	3.7	1.8	2.5*	1.0*
Stomach trouble, N.O.S.	501	100.0	66.5	12.9	5.0	5.7	4.1*	1.4*
Liver condition	411	100.0	61.6	6.3	2.5	9.0	7.8*	10.7

*May be unreliable
Note: N.O.S. = not otherwise specified
Source: *Vital and Health Statistics,* Series 10, No. 115

TABLE 1–6. Selected Chronic Digestive Conditions Reported in Health Interviews and Percentage Distribution of Conditions by Number of Times Doctor Was Seen in Year Prior to Interview: United States, 1975

| CHRONIC CONDITION | CONDITIONS (IN THOUSANDS) | PHYSICIAN VISITS | | | | | |
		Total	None	1	2–4	≥5	Unknown
		Percent distribution					
Ulcer of stomach and duodenum	3,955	100.0	36.1	17.8	26.3	15.8	4.0
Frequent constipation	3,811	100.0	53.1	19.5	26.7	7.8	4.0
Hernia of abdominal cavity	3,725	100.0	35.9	21.6	25.6	12.6	4.2
Functional and symptomatic upper gastrointestinal disorder	3,462	100.0	53.4	17.5	14.8	8.6	5.7
Gallbladder condition	1,625	100.0	32.0	18.7	27.7	17.0	4.7
Gastritis and duodenitis	1,465	100.0	32.8	20.6	27.1	14.9	4.5
Diverticula of intestine	1,323	100.0	42.9	19.4	21.0	13.5	3.2
Chronic enteritis and ulcerative colitis	1,183	100.0	32.5	21.2	23.5	17.3	5.6
Intestinal condition	876	100.0	33.2	24.4	26.0	12.4	3.9
Stomach trouble, N.O.S.	501	100.0	33.2	15.6	24.4	19.2	7.7
Liver condition	411	100.0	26.8	13.6	23.3	31.5	4.7

Note: N.O.S.- = not otherwise specified
Source: *Vital and Health Statistics,* Series 10, No. 115

TABLE 1–7.   Selected Chronic Digestive Conditions Reported in Health Interviews and Percentage of Conditions by Whether Ever Hospitalized, Ever Surgically Treated, or at the Time of Interview under Medical Treatment Recommended by a Doctor: United States, 1975

| | | PERCENTAGE OF CONDITIONS FOR WHICH— | | |
CHRONIC CONDITION	CONDITIONS (IN THOUSANDS)	Ever Hospitalized	Ever Had Surgery	Were Currently Under Treatment or Medication Recommended by a Doctor
		Percent		
Ulcer of stomach and duodenum	3,955	38.3	8.1	65.4
Frequent constipation	3,811	5.4	2.6	52.2
Hernia of abdominal cavity	3,725	31.9	22.8	31.6
Functional and symptomatic upper gastrointestinal disorder	3,462	7.6	1.7	45.8
Gallbladder condition	1,625	42.1	24.9	33.7
Gastritis and duodenitis	1,465	17.8	3.6	59.3
Diverticula of intestine	1,323	29.1	7.5	45.3
Chronic enteritis and ulcerative colitis	1,183	24.8	6.2	47.8
Intestinal condition	876	19.4	5.2	52.6
Stomach trouble, N.O.S.	501	21.2	5.9	49.5
Liver condition	411	41.0	9.4	38.0

Note: N.O.S. = not otherwise specified
Source: *Vital and Health Statistics,* Series 10, No. 115

TABLE 1–8.   Selected Chronic Digestive Conditions Reported in Health Interviews and Percentage Distribution of Conditions by Frequency of Bother: United States, 1975

| | | FREQUENCY OF BOTHER | | | | | |
CHRONIC CONDITION	CONDITIONS (IN THOUSANDS)	Total	All the Time	Some of the Time	Other	Never	Unknown
		Percentage distribution					
Ulcer of stomach and duodenum	3,955	100.0	10.1	75.2	2.0	10.4	2.3
Frequent constipation	3,811	100.0	25.0	67.4	1.1	5.6	0.9
Hernia of abdominal cavity	3,725	100.0	10.6	56.2	1.4	28.9	3.0
Functional and symptomatic upper gastrointestinal disorder	3,462	100.0	11.6	82.8	1.0	2.7	1.9
Gallbladder condition	1,625	100.0	6.5	59.3	1.5	30.0	2.6
Gastritis and duodenitis	1,465	100.0	11.4	78.9	0.7	7.5	1.4
Diverticula of intestine	1,323	100.0	8.9	68.3	1.8	19.8	1.2
Chronic enteritis and ulcerative colitis	1,183	100.0	12.2	75.8	1.2	7.6	3.2
Intestinal condition	876	100.0	8.9	79.9	1.6	6.6	3.1
Stomach trouble, N.O.S.	501	100.0	16.0	71.0	2.4	7.3	3.4
Liver condition	411	100.0	16.3	38.8	2.1	39.5	3.3

Note: N.O.S. = not otherwise specified
Source: *Vital and Health Statistics,* Series 110, No. 115

Subjective complaints of pain or discomfort were reported for selected diseases (Tables 1–8 and 1–9). Frequency of discomfort was highest for constipation followed by unspecified stomach trouble and liver conditions. Intensity was greatest for ulcer, gastritis, enteritis and colitis, and unspecified stomach trouble.

The degree of bother reported is summarized in Table 1–9.

The impact in terms of days of disability, restricted activity, and the seeking of medical attention is summarized in Table 1–10.

TABLE 1–9.   Selected Chronic Digestive Conditions Reported in Health Interviews and Percentage Distribution of Conditions by Degree of Bother: United States, 1975

CHRONIC CONDITION	CONDITIONS (IN THOUSANDS)	Total	DEGREE OF BOTHER						
			Bothered					Not both-ered	Un-known if both-ered
			All	Great deal	Some	Very little	Un-known		
					Percent distribution				
Ulcer of stomach and duodenum	3,955	100.0	87.3	35.1	38.3	12.2	1.8	10.4	2.3
Frequent constipation	3,811	100.0	93.5	27.7	47.2	15.7	2.9	5.6	0.9
Hernia of abdominal cavity	3,725	100.0	68.1	20.7	30.3	15.2	1.9	28.9	3.0
Functional and symptomatic upper gastrointestinal disorder	3,462	100.0	95.4	29.3	51.3	12.5	2.3	2.7	1.9
Gallbladder condition	1,625	100.0	67.4	27.7	27.0	11.1	1.6	30.0	2.6
Gastritis and duodenitis	1,465	100.0	91.0	34.3	40.6	14.2	2.0	7.5	1.4
Diverticula of intestine	1,323	100.0	79.0	25.4	36.2	16.0	1.5	19.8	1.2
Chronic enteritis and ulcerative colitis	1,183	100.0	89.2	34.0	40.0	13.0	2.2	7.6	3.2
Intestinal condition	876	100.0	90.3	35.6	38.2	14.6	2.0	6.6	3.1
Stomach trouble, N.O.S	501	100.0	89.3	34.7	40.9	10.4	3.3	7.3	3.4
Liver condition	411	100.0	57.2	22.7	27.0	7.1	0.4	39.5	3.3

Note: N.O.S. = not otherwise specified
Source: *Vital and Health Statistics*, Series 10, No. 115

TABLE 1–10.   Selected Chronic Digestive Conditions Reported in Health Interviews, Percentage of Conditions by Measures of Impact, and Disability Days per Condition per Year by Type of Disability: United States, 1975

CHRONIC CONDITION	CONDITIONS (IN THOUSANDS)	PERCENT OF CONDITIONS				DISABILITY DAYS			
		Causing Limitation of Activity	With 1 or More Bed-Days in Past Year	With Doctor Ever Seen	With 1 or More Physician Visits in Past Year	Restricted-Activity Days per Condition Per Year	Bed-Days Per Condition Per Year	Bed-Days Per Bed-Disabling Condition Per Year	Work-Loss Days Per Condition Per Year
Ulcer of stomach and duodenum	3,955	13.5	22.7	97.9	59.9	18.0	5.9	26.0	2.2
Frequent constipation	3,811	1.0*	4.9	69.3	43.0	3.6	0.9*	19.0*	0.1*
Hernia of abdominal cavity	3,725	17.6	21.8	96.2	59.9	17.1	4.9	22.6	2.0
Functional and symptomatic upper gastrointestinal disorder	3,462	2.4	8.0	67.0	40.9	9.2	2.3	28.5	0.6*
Gallbladder condition	1,625	9.2	37.4	97.9	63.4	20.0	7.8	20.9	3.2
Gastritis and duodenitis	1,465	3.4	21.3	89.1	62.6	11.9	3.9	18.2	1.7*
Diverticula of intestine	1,323	6.8	16.7	99.2	53.9	12.2	3.6*	21.6*	0.8*
Chronic enteritis and ulcerative colitis	1,183	8.7	21.1	90.4	61.9	13.8	4.5	21.3	1.6*
Intestinal condition	876	4.3	15.4	93.0	62.9	9.7	2.1*	13.4*	0.8*
Stomach trouble, N.O.S.	501	13.2	28.9	85.6	59.1	24.8	11.4	39.2	1.7*
Liver condition	411	27.3	36.3	98.2	68.5	26.6	13.2*	36.3*	2.8*

*May be unreliable
Note: N.O.S. = not otherwise specified
Source: Vital and Health Statistics, Series 10, No. 115

Major Digestive Diseases

2

A peptic ulcer can be either gastric (the lesion is in the stomach) or duodenal (the lesion is in the duodenum, the narrow neck that connects the stomach and the large intestine). Although the exact cause of peptic ulcer is unknown, several aspects of modern life are associated with an exacerbation of ulcer problems. Until the 1970s, men smoked much more than did women. The decline in peptic ulcer disease among men, which is evident since 1960, partly coincides with a decline in smoking.

PEPTIC ULCER

Pain is the chief symptom of peptic ulcer. Yet 15% of sufferers do not experience pain. They are diagnosed from the finding of blood in the stool and low hematocrit levels. The majority with gastric pain often develop it within 4 hours of eating or are awakened by it at night. They find that eating relieves the pain. It may recur for several weeks followed by remission for as long as 3 to 12 months.

Diagnosis is typically made by upper gastrointestinal radiography. More invasive panendoscopy is used to determine whether or not the ulcer is cancerous and in those instances in which scar tissue makes radiography impractical. Treatment still involves bed rest and avoidance of nicotine, caffeine, and alcohol—substances that stimulate stomach acid secretion. Current medical thought does not favor diet modification other than the ingestion of antacids after meals. Although many ulcers treated properly heal within 3 to 6 weeks of medical attention, some patients need to undergo surgical treatment because the ulcer is intractable, causing obstruction, hemorrhage, or perforation.

Newer drugs, such as cimetidine, facilitate healing so the management challenge today is less a question of healing an ulcer than of preventing recurrence in the healed patient. Recent ulcer research shows great promise for both speedy healing and prevention. It involves administering prostaglandins to those who already have an ulcer as well as the ulcer prone.

Prostaglandins, found in all mammalian tissue, are long-chain oxygenated fatty acids derived from arachidonic acid. They not only regulate and inhibit gastric acid secretion but also protect the gastric mucosa. Prostaglandin deficiency is now suspected as a possible cause of gastric hyperacidity and of inflammatory bowel disease. Several prostaglandins have been found to suppress acidity even in the presence of such acid-triggering agents as histamine; stress; reserpine; and nonsteroidal, anti-inflammatory drugs. Low doses of prostaglandins that do not affect other organs can both prevent ulcer formation and heal existing ulcers within 14 days of administration, a record that matches the success of cimetidine.

Prostaglandins can be administered orally. A few nanograms can prevent stomach necrosis ordinarily produced experimentally in animals by ethanol or boiling water. This represents what may be an important breakthrough not only in treatment but in prevention of this sometimes fatal condition.

The peptic ulcer death rate from 1960 through 1984 for subjects by sex, age, and race is summarized in Table 2–1.

Although ulcer is uncommon in children (data not shown in Table 2–1), the health profession is turning its attention to the pediatric form of this condition. In 1979, 17 deaths from duodenal and gastric ulcers were reported for children younger than age 5 years. Seven others occurred in teenagers, age 15 to 19 years.

The duodenal and gastric death rate for populations in several other countries is summarized in Table 2–2. More than a few have rates higher than that of the United States as of the 1980s. The United States has experienced a marked decline in incidence and mortality of peptic ulcer.

Socioeconomic and demographic characteristics of peptic-ulcer sufferers are presented in Table 2–3. Peptic ulcer has long been connected in the lay and scientific populations with stress. The data bear out this supposition (Table 2–3). As expected, people who live alone, who are unemployed, who are separated from spouses,

TABLE 2–1.   Death Rates for Peptic Ulcer, by Age, Race, and Sex; and Corresponding Age-adjusted Rates: United States, 1960–1984 (For 1968–77 rates are based on deaths assigned to category numbers 531–533 of the *Eighth Revision International Classification of Diseases, Adapted for Use in the United States, 1965* [ICDA]; for 1960–67 rates are based on deaths assigned to category numbers 540, 541 of the *Seventh Revision* adopted in 1955)

RACE, SEX, AND YEAR	All Ages	25–34 Years	35–44 Years	45–54 Years	55–64 Years	65–74 Years	75–84 Years	85 Years and Over	Age-Adjusted Rate
Both sexes				*Rate per 100,000 population					
1984	2.8								
1983	2.7								
1982	2.9								
1977*	2.7	0.2	0.7	1.9	4.9	10.5	24.3	46.3	1.8
1976*	3.0	0.3	0.9	2.5	5.6	12.1	25.5	46.5	2.1
1975*	3.2	0.3	0.9	2.5	6.2	12.8	27.5	49.4	2.2
1974*	3.3	0.3	1.1	2.7	7.1	13.6	29.1	50.1	2.4
1973*	3.7	0.4	1.2	3.3	7.6	15.8	30.8	54.2	2.7
1972*,†	3.8	0.4	1.3	3.6	8.0	16.4	31.2	55.2	2.9
1971*	3.9	0.4	1.4	3.9	8.4	16.7	33.1	57.5	3.0
1970*	4.2	0.5	1.4	4.0	9.6	18.0	35.5	59.6	3.2
1969	4.6	0.5	1.8	4.2	10.2	20.1	41.2	64.8	3.6
1968	4.7	0.5	1.7	4.5	10.8	21.5	39.5	69.0	3.7
1967	5.0	0.5	1.8	4.9	11.4	21.5	42.5	79.4	3.9
1966	5.3	0.5	1.9	5.3	11.8	23.8	46.5	79.0	4.2
1965	5.4	0.5	1.9	5.7	12.6	23.9	47.2	81.2	4.3
1964	5.7	0.6	2.2	5.9	13.6	25.8	50.8	85.2	4.6
1963	6.5	0.8	2.5	7.1	14.8	29.5	56.6	92.9	5.2
1962	6.6	0.7	2.6	7.0	15.4	30.6	57.3	94.6	5.4
1961	6.3	0.8	2.4	7.4	15.1	29.4	53.5	82.8	5.2
1960	6.3	0.7	2.5	7.3	15.7	29.9	53.6	77.9	5.2

White, male

Year									
1982	3.0	0.3	0.8	2.7	7.0	16.2	35.8	63.3	2.6
1977*	3.5	0.2	1.0	3.3	8.1	18.8	39.8	68.1	3.0
1976*	3.9	0.3	1.1	3.3	8.6	20.9	42.1	74.5	3.3
1975*	4.2								
1974*	4.4	0.4	1.3	3.8	10.1	20.9	45.8	74.8	3.6
1973*	5.0	0.3	1.4	4.4	11.6	25.5	48.3	78.3	4.0
1972*†	5.2	0.4	1.7	5.0	11.5	25.9	49.3	88.9	4.3
1971*	5.4	0.4	1.7	5.2	12.9	27.0	51.6	89.5	4.5
1970*	5.9	0.5	1.7	5.6	14.9	28.9	56.2	88.3	4.8
1969	6.5	0.7	2.2	6.3	15.8	32.4	63.8	94.7	5.4
1968	6.8	0.6	2.0	6.4	16.7	35.3	63.7	102.3	5.6
1967	7.3	0.6	2.3	6.8	18.6	36.6	66.5	121.2	6.0
1966	7.7	0.6	2.5	7.5	18.5	39.4	76.1	119.8	6.4
1965	8.0	0.6	2.5	8.1	20.6	40.7	75.6	128.7	6.8
1964	8.6	0.7	2.9	8.4	22.3	43.7	80.5	137.2	7.3
1963*	9.8	1.0	3.3	10.7	24.0	50.2	91.9	145.2	8.3
1962*	10.0	0.9	3.6	10.4	24.7	51.5	92.4	144.3	8.4
1961	9.7	1.1	3.5	11.0	25.1	49.5	86.3	129.2	8.3
1960	10.0	1.0	3.6	11.3	26.8	50.4	88.5	120.9	8.5

All other, male

Year								
1982	2.4	0.8	3.9	10.1	14.5	24.4	26.4	3.0
1977*	2.6	1.5	6.3	9.0	18.9	30.8	42.6	3.7
1976*	3.3	0.8	5.7	11.5	19.0	31.7	35.9	3.8
1975*	3.3							
1974*	3.6	0.9	6.7	12.5	22.1	26.4	42.1	4.1
1973*	4.2	1.4	7.0	13.3	24.9	38.5	35.8	4.9
1972*†	4.7	1.2	9.7	16.9	27.3	35.4	27.5	5.5
1971*	4.4	2.1	9.9	13.6	21.3	33.7	30.6	5.1
1970*	4.6	1.7	9.4	14.1	26.8	40.4	23.5	5.4
1969	5.0	1.3	8.9	17.6	27.0	53.7	22.7	5.8
1968	5.5	2.4	10.7	19.3	32.3	33.3	39.0	6.5
1967	5.4	1.5	12.1	18.4	25.1	47.8	61.5	6.3
1966	6.0	1.4	12.1	22.4	33.3	47.5	61.1	7.0
1965	5.6	1.6	12.9	19.4	28.2	47.7	38.2	6.6
1964	6.2	1.5	13.2	24.1	33.8	48.3	46.9	7.3
1963‡	6.8	2.2	14.0	25.1	37.2	47.9	37.9	7.8
1962‡	7.1	3.2	13.8	26.1	40.3	41.0	58.6	8.2
1961	6.7	3.3	14.8	22.0	38.1	45.9	56.7	7.8
1960	6.9	2.2	15.0	23.8	38.7	40.7	44.6	7.8

TABLE 2–1. (Continued)

RACE, SEX, AND YEAR	All Ages	25–34 Years	35–44 Years	45–54 Years	55–64 Years	65–74 Years	75–84 Years	85 Years and Over	Age-Adjusted Rate
				Rate per 100,000 population					
White female									
1977*	2.3	0.1	0.5	0.9	2.7	6.2	18.1	42.3	1.2
1976*	2.3	0.1	0.4	1.4	3.3	7.0	17.7	39.8	1.3
1975*	2.4	0.2	0.4	1.5	3.7	6.7	19.5	40.8	1.4
1974*	2.5	0.2	0.5	1.4	4.2	7.9	20.6	41.3	1.5
1973*	2.7	0.3	0.8	1.8	4.0	8.4	20.8	45.6	1.6
1972*†	2.7	0.2	0.4	1.7	4.5	9.2	20.9	43.4	1.6
1971*	2.8	0.2	0.7	2.0	4.1	9.2	22.6	46.5	1.7
1970*	2.9	0.2	0.8	2.1	4.8	10.0	23.6	49.3	1.9
1969	3.1	0.3	1.0	1.9	4.9	10.8	27.1	54.2	2.0
1968	3.1	0.2	0.8	2.4	5.1	11.0	25.2	54.8	2.0
1967	3.1	0.2	0.9	2.6	4.8	10.6	27.3	60.9	2.0
1966	3.3	0.3	0.9	2.5	5.4	11.8	28.1	61.1	2.2
1965	3.2	0.3	1.0	2.8	5.2	11.4	28.9	60.9	2.2
1964	3.3	0.3	1.1	2.8	5.3	12.0	31.6	60.7	2.3
1963‡	3.7	0.3	1.3	3.1	5.7	13.5	34.5	70.1	2.5
1962‡	3.8	0.3	1.2	3.3	6.1	14.1	34.9	71.7	2.6
1961	3.4	0.3	1.1	3.3	5.7	13.2	31.7	58.6	2.4
1960	3.3	0.3	1.0	3.0	5.5	13.1	30.4	57.3	2.4

All other, female

1977*	1.4	0.3	0.8	1.3	3.9	6.5	15.2	21.2
1976*	1.4	0.4	0.9	2.3	3.3	7.4	13.0	16.5
1975*	1.6	0.2	1.0	2.4	4.2	8.0	14.1	21.8
1974*	1.4	0.3	1.2	2.0	3.7	8.7	9.4	20.6
1973*	1.5	0.5	1.0	2.5	3.8	7.0	12.7	27.3
1972*†	1.6	0.7	1.9	3.5	3.9	6.7	13.5	12.2
1971*	1.8	0.6	1.4	3.3	5.6	8.6	14.8	10.5
1970*	1.8	0.6	1.5	3.0	6.9	7.1	9.9	24.2
1969	2.1	0.7	2.4	2.8	5.6	11.5	19.0	30.8
1968	2.1	0.5	2.6	2.9	6.7	9.3	15.9	44.3
1967	2.2	0.7	2.2	3.1	6.6	8.1	20.3	35.1
1966	2.3	0.4	2.1	5.6	6.1	10.8	13.1	28.3
1965	2.2	0.5	1.9	4.1	7.2	9.0	19.2	24.5
1964	2.6	1.1	3.0	5.8	6.1	10.2	20.0	33.3
1963‡	2.5	0.9	1.9	4.9	8.8	13.0	13.5	31.0
1962‡	2.3	0.4	2.4	3.6	9.6	11.0	15.8	30.0
1961	2.5	0.7	1.7	5.2	9.2	11.6	18.3	40.0
1960	2.2	0.8	2.3	4.2	6.6	11.0	14.3	19.9

*Excludes deaths of nonresidents of the United States
†Based on a 50% sample of deaths
‡Figures by race exclude data for residents of New Jersey because this state did not require reporting of the item for these years
Source: *Vital and Health Statistics*, Series 17, No. 20

TABLE 2–2.   Mortality Rates for Various Countries for Peptic Ulcer by Latest Reported Year

COUNTRY	RATE (per 100,000)	YEAR
Costa Rica	1.8	1981
Guatemala	1.6	1980
Chile	2.7	1980
Israel	2.0	1980
Japan	4.7	1980
Kuwait	0.5	1979
Austria	9.0	1981
Bulgaria	4.6	1981
France	4.4	1981
Greece	2.7	1981
Hungary	10.2	1980
Poland	5.8	1980
United Kingdom, England, Wales	9.0	1981
Australia	4.8	1980
United States	2.5	1980*

*The year reported is 1980 for purposes of comparability with other rates presented.
Source: *U.N. Demographic Yearbook*, 1982

who earn less than $5,000 annually, who have less education, and who live outside urban areas and are more likely to be poor are more susceptible to ulcers than other segments of the population.

The prevalence of ulcers has been declining in both men and women since the 1960s. Figure 2–1 shows how significant that decline is in the number of people age 45 to 64 years who were hospitalized for peptic ulcer between 1965 and 1980. The largest decreases occurred between 1965 and 1970 when the first major campaigns against smoking were in vogue and again between 1975 and 1980.

FREQUENT CONSTIPATION

Constipation is typically defined as having a bowel movement less often than every other day or passing stools that are small or excessively dry. The possible causes of constipation include some systemic diseases, such as diabetes mellitus, hypothyroidism, and hyperparathyroidism or exposure to toxic substances, such as lead opiates and aluminum hydroxide. Local disorders, such as weak abdominal muscles, restriction of the anal canal, and sacral cord disease may also cause constipation. A low-fiber diet also contributes to constipation.

FIG. 2–1. Rates per 1,000 population for patients aged 45–64 years discharged from short-stay hospitals with a diagnosis of gastric, duodenal, and other unspecified peptic ulcers, by sex: United States, 1965, 1970, 1975, 1980

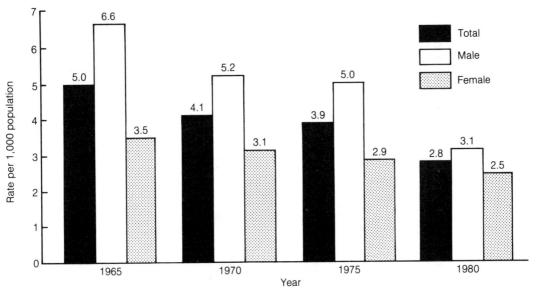

Source: *Vital and Health Statistics*, Series 13, No. 74

The general public as well as the medical profession have long known that fibrous foods can alleviate constipation. A major area of study today concerns the efficacy of a high fiber diet in both relieving constipation and preventing intestinal diseases, including colon cancer.

There are many different types of fiber, both soluble and insoluble, and their health value varies widely. While scientists have not yet drawn definitive conclusions regarding the benefits of dietary fiber, convincing research does indicate that some types of fiber may help to lower cholesterol levels while others may help to protect against colon cancer. Some researchers warn that high fiber diets tend to deplete the body's supply of trace minerals, particularly zinc, since these minerals bind with the fiber. Others believe that this issue is of practical relevance only to those consuming a nutritionally marginal diet such as teenagers, the elderly and the poor.

The initial hypothesis that high-fiber diets promoted intestinal wellbeing was suggested by observing natives of South Africa. The rural blacks of this region eat diets composed mostly of vegetables with dietary-fiber contents of more than 50 g daily. These Africans

TABLE 2–3. Number and Rate per 1,000 Population of Ulcers of Stomach and Duodenum Reported in Health Interviews, by Age and Selected Characteristics: United States, 1975 (data are based on household interviews of the civilian noninstitutionalized population)

CHARACTERISTIC	ALL AGES	UNDER 45 YEARS Total	UNDER 45 YEARS 17–44 Years	45–64 YEARS	65 YEARS AND OVER	ALL AGES	UNDER 45 YEARS Total	UNDER 45 YEARS 17–44 Years	45–64 YEARS	65 YEARS AND OVER
	Number of conditions in thousands					Rate per 1,000 population				
Total	3,955	1,846	1,773	1,453	656	18.9	12.8	21.4	33.7	30.8
Sex										
Male	2,091	962	920	805	324	20.7	13.4	23.0	39.2	36.9
Female	1,863	885	853	647	331	17.2	12.1	19.9	28.7	26.5
Race										
White	3,542	1,624	1,560	1,312	605	19.5	13.1	21.7	33.9	31.3
All other	413	222	214	140	50	15.2	10.7	19.9	31.6	25.7
Black	385	205	196	130	50	15.8	11.0	20.9	32.5	27.4
Usual activity status										
School age (6–16 years)	71	71	...	...	...	1.7	1.7	...	...	...
Usually working (17 years and over)	1,994	1,172	1,172	762	60	25.1	23.4	23.5	28.2	24.3
Usually keeping house (female, 17 years and over)	1,109	419	419	401	289	27.6	23.6	23.7	33.0	28.0
Retired (45 years and over)	458	...	...	186	272	46.8	...	...	79.0	36.5
Other activity (17 years and over)	317	180	180	104	33*	18.2	12.0	12.0	70.4	31.6*
Marital status										
Married	2,820	1,298	1,298	1,152	369	28.8	25.0	25.0	33.5	32.0
Formerly married	730	220	220	248	262	34.6	35.3	35.3	38.7	30.9
Widowed	370	15*	15*	128	226	32.1	30.9*	30.9*	37.9	29.5
Separated	123	63	63	49	11*	37.3	29.6	29.6	53.2	45.3*
Divorced	238	141	141	71	26*	37.9	39.0	39.0	33.6	46.8*
Never married	331	255	255	52	24*	11.7	10.4	10.4	22.7	18.5*

Employment status										
In the labor force (17 years and over)	2,199	1,303	1,303	813	83	24.1	21.8	21.8	28.7	27.6
Employed	1,940	1,128	1,128	738	74	23.3	21.0	21.0	27.6	26.4
Unemployed	259	176	176	75	9*	32.8	29.0	29.0	46.3	42.9*
Not in the labor force (17 years and over)	1,682	470	470	640	572	30.0	20.5	20.5	43.3	31.3
Living arrangements										
Living alone	475	120	120	170	185	31.0	22.4	22.6	40.8	31.8
Living with nonrelatives	79	65	65	9*	5*	21.6	22.8	23.0	18.4*	15.9*
Living with spouse	2,783	1,271	1,271	1,147	366	28.7	24.8	24.8	33.6	32.1
Living with other relatives	617	391	318	127	99	6.6	4.6	13.7	29.6	26.3
Family income										
Less than $5,000	923	307	300	282	334	29.1	17.0	29.5	53.1	40.0
$5,000–$9,999	984	464	458	370	150	21.7	15.2	26.8	42.4	25.4
$10,000–$14,999	797	461	440	272	64	16.9	12.9	21.6	29.6	29.9
$15,000 or more	1,009	535	500	420	54	14.4	10.4	16.5	26.6	22.0
Education of head of family										
Less than 12 years	1,966	656	628	821	489	25.7	14.8	27.1	43.6	37.0
12 years	1,118	683	652	363	72	16.4	13.3	22.1	27.9	17.9
13–15 years	454	273	268	132	48	15.9	12.3	19.2	28.3	28.4
16 years or more	366	220	210	113	33*	11.2	8.8	13.8	19.4	17.8*
Place of Residence										
SMSA	2,494	1,212	1,156	933	349	17.4	12.1	19.8	31.4	25.9
Central city	1,079	513	498	399	167	17.5	12.2	20.1	30.8	25.0
Outside central city	1,415	699	658	534	182	17.2	12.0	19.6	31.8	26.7
Outside SMSA	1,461	634	617	520	307	22.3	14.3	25.2	38.9	39.4
Nonfarm	1,350	598	583	463	288	23.0	14.9	26.2	40.0	41.5
Farm	111	35	36	56	19*	16.5	8.9	15.9	31.1	22.1*
Region										
Northeast	772	321	311	295	157	15.7	9.8	16.5	27.2	29.1
North Central	1,024	470	448	398	156	18.3	12.1	20.1	35.6	26.6
South	1,311	600	571	470	241	19.6	12.9	21.7	34.9	36.0
West	848	455	444	291	102	22.8	17.3	29.1	38.4	30.5

*May be unreliable
Source: *Vital and Health Statistics*, Series 10, No. 115

TABLE 2–4. Number and Rate per 1,000 Population of Frequent Constipation Reported in Health Interviews, by Age and Selected Characteristics: United States, 1975 (data are based on household interviews of the civilian noninstitutionalized population)

CHARACTERISTIC	Number of conditions in thousands					Rate per 1,000 population				
	ALL AGES	UNDER 45 YEARS Total	17–44 Years	45–64 YEARS	65 YEARS AND OVER	ALL AGES	UNDER 45 YEARS Total	17–44 Years	45–64 YEARS	65 YEARS AND OVER
Total	3,811	1,367	1,049	1,015	1,429	18.2	9.4	12.7	23.6	67.1
Sex										
Male	902	298	166	221	383	8.9	4.2	4.2	10.8	43.6
Female	2,909	1,069	883	793	1,046	26.9	14.6	20.6	35.2	83.6
Race										
White	3,180	1,050	813	864	1,266	17.5	8.5	11.3	22.3	65.5
All other	630	317	235	151	163	23.2	15.2	21.8	34.1	83.6
Black	589	294	216	141	154	24.1	15.8	23.1	35.2	84.3
Usual Activity Status										
School age (6-16 years)	154	154	...	...	...	3.6	3.6	...	...	...
Usually working (17 years and over)	961	516	516	377	68	12.1	10.3	10.3	14.0	27.5
Usually keeping house (female, 17 years and over)	1,791	432	430	493	865	44.6	24.4	24.3	40.6	83.9
Retired (45 years and over)	438	...	...	82	356	44.7	...	...	34.8	47.8
Other activity (17 years and over)	300	103	103	61	136	17.2	6.9	6.9	41.3	130.1
Marital status										
Married	1,921	670	670	660	591	19.6	12.9	11.6	19.2	51.3
Formerly married	1,160	138	138	285	737	55.0	22.1	22.1	44.5	87.0
Widowed	874	12*	12*	179	682	75.8	24.7*	24.7*	53.0	88.9
Separated	109	54	54	37	18*	33.1	25.4	25.4	40.2	74.1*
Divorced	177	71	71	69	37	28.2	19.6	19.6	32.7	66.5
Never married	412	241	241	69	101	14.6	9.8	9.8	30.1	77.8

Employment Status									
In the labor force (17 years and over)	1,135	604	604	427	105	12.5	10.1	10.1	15.1	34.9
Employed	1,013	529	529	389	95	12.2	9.8	9.8	14.6	33.9
Unemployed	123	75	75	38	10*	15.6	12.3	12.3	23.5	47.6*
Not in the labor force (17 years and over)	2,357	445	445	588	1,324	42.1	19.4	19.4	39.8	72.4
Living Arrangements									
Living alone	838	84	84	212	542	54.6	15.7	15.8	50.8	93.1
Living with nonrelatives	82	35	35	24*	23*	22.4	12.3	12.4	49.0*	73.0*
Living with spouse	1,884	656	656	655	573	19.4	12.8	12.8	19.2	50.3
Living with other relatives	1,007	592	274	124	291	10.8	7.0	11.8	28.9	77.4
Family income									
Less than $5,000	1,373	283	224	298	791	43.2	15.7	22.0	56.1	94.7
$5,000-$9,999	922	343	266	257	322	20.4	11.2	15.5	29.4	54.4
$10,000-$14,999	509	264	210	160	86	10.8	7.4	10.3	17.4	40.2
$15,000 or more	701	395	293	223	84	10.0	7.7	9.7	14.1	34.3
Education of Head of Family									
Less than 12 years	2,039	456	348	581	1,002	26.6	10.3	15.0	30.8	75.8
12 years	908	459	352	250	198	13.3	9.0	12.0	19.2	49.1
13-15 years	411	222	177	69	119	14.4	10.0	12.7	14.8	70.3
16 years or more	376	198	153	97	80	11.5	7.9	10.1	16.7	43.2
Place of Residence									
SMSA	2,492	1,000	769	636	856	17.3	10.0	13.2	21.4	63.4
Central city	1,272	525	401	298	449	20.7	12.5	16.2	23.0	67.3
Outside central city	1,221	475	368	338	407	14.9	8.1	11.0	20.1	59.7
Outside SMSA	1,318	367	280	379	573	20.1	8.3	11.4	28.3	73.5
Nonfarm	1,231	358	272	333	539	21.0	8.9	12.2	28.8	77.7
Farm	87	8*	8*	45	33*	13.0	2.0*	3.6*	25.0	38.4*
Region									
Northeast	822	334	258	187	302	16.7	10.2	13.7	17.2	56.0
North Central	791	284	229	194	313	14.2	7.3	10.3	17.3	53.4
South	1,472	478	350	422	572	22.0	10.2	13.3	31.3	85.5
West	726	271	212	212	242	19.5	10.3	13.9	28.0	72.4

*May be unreliable
Source: *Vital and Health Statistics*, Series 10, No. 115

are remarkably free of polyps, colon cancer, appendicitis, and diverticulosis. They also develop fewer hiatal hernias and less heart disease and diabetes. Natives who moved to urban areas and assumed a more Western diet have begun to experience many of the diseases just mentioned at rates similar to those in Western industrialized countries. Their Western way of life is also more sedentary. Some believe that their habit of walking great distances in their rural setting plays a major role in their health, independent of fiber.

Although the benefits of the various types of fiber have not been scientifically confirmed, current research and the initial epidemiologic evidence from South Africa suggests that a high fiber diet may inhibit certain diseases and colon syndromes. The National Cancer Institute (NCI) has recommended that Americans increase their dietary fiber from the current average of 15 g to 30 g per day.

Those investigators testing the hypothesis that high-fiber diets are beneficial theorize that the greater bulk or weight of high-fiber diet stools may dilute the concentrations of toxic substances in fecal matter that ordinarily lead to irritation and ultimately cancer of the colon. They also suspect that the greater speed with which the stool is processed and expelled may provide protection since toxic substances are in shorter contact with intestinal mucosa. Research continues.

Many of the demographic characteristics associated with peptic ulcer also correlate with chronic constipation. One exception relates to women with low incomes. Those who are separated from spouses are more likely than low-income, separated men to be constipated. Residents of the South and West reported more constipation than inhabitants of other parts of the country even when the ages of regional populations were taken into account.

A direct relationship exists between age and constipation: the condition is more common as one grows older. The reported constipation rate for persons younger than age 17 years is 5.1 per 1,000. But the rate for those older than 65 years is 67.1 per 1,000. The full profile of the relationship between age and constipation is seen in Table 2–4.

The most common disability related to constipation is hemorrhoids. Chronic constipation causes hemorrhoids that are thought to afflict 70% of the population. Based on the results of government studies, the finding suggests that constipation may be greatly under-reported because it is generally a nonserious condition that does not cause disability. People may report a hemorrhoid disorder but not constipation because the former causes more discomfort than the latter.

HERNIA

Generally, a hernia is the rupture and protrusion of an organ or component through the boundaries that typically confine it. A hiatus hernia is a protrusion of part of the stomach through the esophageal hiatus above the diaphragm. An inguinal hernia is a protrusion of the sac containing a loop of bowel at the inguinal opening.

The cause is often muscle strain as when one improperly lifts a heavy load. But hernia can also be caused by the strain of coughing, obesity, pregnancy, or muscular weakness after a lengthy illness. It may also result from the strain of constipation. The danger of hiatus hernia is the reflux of stomach acid and pepsin, irritating the esophageal mucosa. This in turn can cause heartburn, internal bleeding, and anemia. Definitive diagnosis is done by esophagoscopy, which will show esophageal inflammation. Radiographic examination of the stomach and small intestine can also furnish diagnostic information.

The 5-year mortality from hernia (1980–1984) is shown in Table 2–5.

The demographic characteristics of those who develop hernias are shown in Table 2–6. In those patients younger than age 45 years, income is not related to hernia. But in older people, family income is inversely related to incidence. Hernia is also more common among whites than non-whites.

FUNCTIONAL AND SYMPTOMATIC UPPER GASTROINTESTINAL DISORDERS

Prominent among these disorders is upper gastrointestinal (GI) bleeding caused by gastritis, gastric varices (dilation of a vein), a

TABLE 2–5. Mortality Data from Hernia, United States, 1980–84

	1980	1981	1982	1983	1984
Number	6,930	5,430	4,980	5,150	5,360
Rate per 100,000	2.5	3.0	2.2	2.2	2.3

Source: *Monthly Vital Statistics Report*, 32,33; numbers 9,12,13; September 1984, December 1984, March 1985

TABLE 2–6. Number and Rate per 1,000 Population of Hernias of Abdominal Cavity Reported in Health Interviews, by Age and Selected Characteristics: United States, 1975 (data are based on interviews of the civilian non-institutionalized population)

CHARACTERISTIC	Number and conditions in thousands					Rate per 1,000 population				
	ALL AGES	UNDER 45 YEARS Total	UNDER 45 YEARS 17–44 Years	45–64 YEARS	65 YEARS AND OVER	ALL AGES	UNDER 45 YEARS Total	UNDER 45 YEARS 17–44 Years	45–64 YEARS	65 YEARS AND OVER
Total	3,725	924	710	1,477	1,324	17.8	6.4	8.6	34.3	62.2
Sex:										
Male	1,954	545	409	784	625	19.4	7.6	10.2	38.2	71.2
Female	1,771	378	301	693	699	16.4	5.2	7.0	30.7	55.9
Race:										
White	3,496	801	657	1,416	1,279	19.2	6.5	9.1	36.6	66.1
All other	229	123	53	61	45	8.4	5.9	4.9	13.8	23.1
Black	215	113	48	61	41	8.8	6.1	5.1	15.2	22.4
Usual Activity Status:										
School age (6–16 years)	99	99	...	...	...	2.3	2.3	...	...	...
Usually working (17 years and over)	1,349	482	482	754	113	17.0	9.6	9.6	27.9	45.7
Usually keeping house (female, 17 years and over)	1,221	156	156	460	605	30.4	8.8	8.8	37.9	58.7
Retired (45 years and over)	725	...	...	173	552	74.0	...	...	73.5	74.2
Other activity (17 years and over)	211	68	68	88	55	12.1	4.6	4.6	59.5	52.6
Marital Status:										
Married	2,458	546	546	1,176	736	25.1	10.5	10.5	34.2	63.9
Formerly married	842	91	91	220	530	39.9	14.6	14.6	34.2	62.6
Widowed	584	7*	7*	108	469	50.6	14.4*	14.4*	32.0	61.2
Separated	74	25*	25*	37	13*	22.5	11.7*	11.7*	40.2	53.5*
Divorced	183	60	60	75	49	29.1	16.6	16.6	35.5	88.1
Never married	212	73	73	81	58	7.5	3.0	3.0	35.3	44.7

Employment Status:									
In the labor force (17 years and over)	1,466	540	540	776	149	16.1	9.0	9.0	27.4	49.5
Employed	1,341	487	487	719	134	16.1	9.1	9.1	26.9	47.9
Unemployed	125	53	53	57	15*	15.8	8.7	8.7	35.2	71.4*
Not in the labor force (17 years and over)	2,046	169	169	701	1,175	36.5	7.4	7.4	47.5	64.3
Living Arrangements:									
Living alone	604	33*	33*	168	403	39.4	6.2*	6.2*	40.3	69.2
Living with nonrelatives	42	16*	16*	8*	18*	11.5	5.6*	5.7*	16.3*	57.1*
Living with spouse	2,445	544	544	1,170	731	25.2	10.6	10.6	34.3	64.2
Living with other relatives	635	331	118	131	172	6.8	3.9	5.1	30.5	45.7
Family Income:									
Less than $5,000	959	106	78	273	581	30.2	5.9	7.7	51.4	69.5
$5,000–$9,999	892	212	158	308	372	19.7	6.9	9.2	35.3	62.9
$10,000–$14,999	626	221	170	280	125	13.3	6.2	8.3	30.5	58.5
$15,000 or more	970	349	276	510	111	13.9	6.8	9.1	32.3	45.3
Education of Head of Family:									
Less than 12 years	1,834	283	211	687	864	24.0	6.4	9.1	36.5	65.4
12 years	978	308	245	420	250	14.3	6.0	8.3	32.3	62.0
13–15 years	406	142	113	167	96	14.2	6.4	8.1	35.8	56.7
16 years or more	452	182	135	179	90	13.8	7.2	8.9	30.8	48.6
Place of Residence:									
SMSA	2,371	597	448	954	819	16.5	5.9	7.7	32.1	60.7
Central city	1,006	241	187	402	363	16.3	5.7	7.6	31.1	54.4
Outside central city	1,365	356	260	552	456	16.6	6.1	7.7	32.9	66.9
Outside SMSA	1,354	326	262	523	505	20.7	7.4	10.7	39.1	64.8
Nonfarm	1,206	295	236	460	451	20.5	7.3	10.6	39.7	65.0
Farm	148	31*	26*	63	54	22.1	7.7*	11.8*	35.0	62.9
Region:									
Northeast	924	233	178	360	332	18.8	7.1	9.4	33.1	61.6
North Central	895	239	183	318	338	16.0	6.2	8.2	28.4	57.6
South	1,243	289	214	523	431	18.6	6.2	8.1	38.8	64.4
West	662	163	135	277	223	17.8	6.2	8.9	36.5	66.7

*May be unreliable

Source: *Vital and Health Statistics*, Series 10, No. 115

Mallory-Weiss tear, or esophagitis. Ulcers, which have been discussed separately in a previous section of this chapter, may also cause GI bleeding.

Diagnosis of upper GI bleeding can be made in part by a careful history-taking. The patient may indicate alcohol abuse, long-term or heavy ingestion of aspirin, or a formerly treated ulcer. When blood loss is massive, cardiac output may decrease, blood pressure may drop, and the pulse may be rapid. Mental confusion may occur as hemorrhage continues, resulting in impaired perfusion of the brain.

The annual mortality rate for upper GI bleeding is about 11.5 per 100,000. New hospital admissions total 250,000 yearly, or 115 per 100,000. Those who are susceptible to upper GI bleeding are profiled in Table 2–7. As with other digestive diseases, upper GI disorders are more common among the divorced than the never married or currently married until age 65 years. They are also more common among those living alone, the old, and those earning less than $5,000 per year.

Diagnosis of upper GI bleeding is often made by endoscopy, barium studies, or angiography if other means fail to provide enough information. Locating the bleeding lesion is especially important when surgical treatment is contemplated. Inappropriate procedures are to be avoided when bleeding varices and diffuse gastritis can be ruled out. Controversy surrounds the use of endoscopy. But studies indicate that single-contrast, upper GI series are about one-half as accurate as endoscopy in locating upper GI bleeding. Double-contrast techniques, however, approach the accuracy of endoscopy. Generally, barium studies exclude the possibility of endoscopy or angiography as a follow-up by obscuring the field. They also make surgical repair more difficult in some instances or require repeated radiation exposure when large volumes of blood dilute the barium. Angiography is typically not as accurate as endoscopy. But radionuclide scanning with technetium or tagged RBCs is a newer noninvasive technique. It is currently undergoing evaluation as a diagnostic tool.

Endoscopy is usually indicated when a patient is cooperative and has had continuous or recurrent bleeding during hospitalization without a clear diagnosis. Complications have been noted not only in patients with heart, lung, renal, and liver diseases but also in those receiving immunosuppressive drugs. Resuscitation facilities should be in place in the event of cardiac arrhythmia, hypotension, or hypoxemia. Aspiration is common and more serious when endoscopy is performed during active upper GI bleeding. The most common side effects are cardiopulmonary. They ensue from the procedure or from premedication. Thrombophlebitis may occur after I.V. administration of medication.

Treatment of upper GI bleeding must be prompt, beginning with isotonic saline administration, blood typing, and testing the patient for blood count, liver function, serum electrolyte level, urea, creatinine, glucose, and prothrombin time. If the patient's hematocrit falls below 30% and if resting blood pressure is less than 100/60 mm Hg with a heart rate of more than 100 beats per minute, a blood transfusion is usually given. Of these indicators, the hematocrit is the least reliable, failing to fall in some cases of severe hemorrhage and being low in others when hemorrhage is no longer a problem.

CHOLELITHIASIS (GALLBLADDER)

Gallbladder disease is marked primarily by the formation of either cholesterol or pigment stones. Cholesterol stones constitute the majority of stones. They form when the cholesterol concentration in bile is disproportionate to bile acid and lecithin, which ordinarily dissolve cholesterol and insoluble bile constituents.

If cholesterol or bilirubin remain undissolved in bile, they can precipitate out as stones. When undetected, they are called "silent stones." The stones may remain in the gallbladder or pass out of it, obstructing a main bile duct and causing jaundice.

Recent research has determined that some people who form gallstones also form cholesterol crystals more quickly than those who do not. And investigators are now looking for an agent that will inhibit this process. Many of the 8 out of 1,000 people who suffer from gallstones are asymptomatic. Symptoms often begin when a stone enters the cystic duct, a condition called acute cholecystitis. The symptoms include steady pain in the right upper quadrant, nausea, vomiting, fever, jaundice, decreased bowel sounds, and a palpable gallbladder.

Diagnosis, which depends on history and physical findings, can be facilitated by radiographic studies. At least 20% of cholesterol stones and 80% of pigment stones are opaque on routine abdominal pictures. An I.V. cholangiogram can facilitate a diagnosis of acute cholecystitis as can abdominal ultrasound. Ultrasound is particularly useful since it does not expose the patient to radiation.

Surgical removal is a recommended treatment although the elderly and diabetic are prone to complications. A welcome alter-

TABLE 2-7. Number and Rate per 1,000 Population of Functional and Symptomatic Upper Gastrointestinal Disorders Reported in Health Interviews, by Age and Selected Characteristics: United States, 1975 (data are based on household interviews of the civilian noninstitutionalized population)

CHARACTERISTIC	Number of conditions in thousands					Rate per 1,000 population				
	ALL AGES	UNDER 45 YEARS Total	UNDER 45 YEARS 17–44 Years	45–64 YEARS	65 YEARS AND OVER	ALL AGES	UNDER 45 YEARS Total	UNDER 45 YEARS 17–44 Years	45–64 YEARS	65 YEARS AND OVER
Total	3,462	1,373	1,296	1,269	820	16.6	9.5	15.7	29.4	38.5
Sex:										
Male	1,747	765	729	654	328	17.3	10.7	18.2	31.8	37.4
Female	1,715	608	568	615	492	15.9	8.3	13.3	27.3	39.3
Race:										
White	2,997	1,155	1,093	1,109	734	16.5	9.3	15.2	28.7	38.0
All other	465	219	203	160	87	17.1	10.5	18.9	36.1	44.6
Black	431	200	188	147	84	17.7	10.8	20.1	36.7	46.0
Usual Activity Status:										
School age (6–16 years)	57	57	...	...	...	1.3	1.3	...	...	...
Usually working (17 years and over)	1,625	883	883	676	67	20.4	17.6	17.7	25.0	27.1
Usually keeping house (female, 17 years and over)	1,103	288	288	389	425	27.5	16.2	16.3	32.1	41.2
Retired (45 years and over)	399	...	...	113	286	40.7	...	...	48.0	38.4
Other activity (17 years and over)	257	126	126	89	42	14.7	8.4	8.4	60.2	40.2
Marital Status:										
Married	2,337	980	980	975	382	23.9	18.9	18.9	28.3	33.2
Formerly married	766	148	148	232	386	36.3	23.8	23.8	36.2	45.6
Widowed	479	9*	9*	131	339	41.5	18.6*	18.6*	38.8	44.2
Separated	122	63	63	39	20*	37.0	29.6	29.6	42.3	82.3*
Divorced	165	76	76	62	28*	26.3	21.0	21.0	29.4	50.4*
Never married	283	169	169	63	52	10.0	6.9	6.9	27.5	40.1

Employment Status:									
In the labor force (17 years and over)	1,788	977	977	735	76	19.6	16.3	16.3	26.0	25.2
Employed	1,609	867	867	670	72	19.3	16.1	16.1	25.1	25.7
Unemployed	179	110	110	65	3*	22.6	18.1	18.1	40.1	14.3*
Not in the labor force (17 years and over)	1,598	319	319	534	745	28.5	13.9	13.9	36.1	40.8
Living Arrangements:									
Living alone	584	92	92	184	308	38.1	17.2	17.3	44.1	52.9
Living with nonrelatives	66	40	40	17*	9*	18.0	14.0	14.1	34.7*	28.6*
Living with spouse	2,302	966	966	964	371	23.8	18.8	18.8	28.2	32.6
Living with other relatives	512	276	199	104	131	5.5	3.2	8.6	24.2	34.8
Family Income:									
Less than $5,000	958	203	184	290	465	30.2	11.2	18.1	54.6	55.6
$5,000–$9,999	821	333	313	296	192	18.1	10.9	18.3	33.9	32.4
$10,000–$14,999	624	357	346	241	27*	13.2	10.0	17.0	26.2	12.6*
$15,000 or more	820	422	398	325	74	11.7	8.2	13.2	20.6	30.2
Education of Head of Family:									
Less than 12 years	1,687	404	371	694	589	22.0	9.1	16.0	36.8	44.6
12 years	973	491	470	349	134	14.3	9.6	16.0	26.8	33.2
13–15 years	378	228	215	106	44	13.2	10.2	15.4	22.7	26.0
16 years or more	396	244	234	105	47	12.1	9.7	15.4	18.1	25.4
Place of Residence:									
SMSA	2,204	936	875	789	480	15.3	9.3	15.0	26.5	35.6
Central city	1,027	428	409	364	235	16.7	10.2	16.5	28.1	35.2
Outside central city	1,177	508	465	425	245	14.3	8.7	13.9	25.3	35.9
Outside SMSA	1,259	438	422	480	341	19.2	9.9	17.3	35.9	43.8
Nonfarm	1,139	426	412	412	301	19.4	10.6	18.5	35.6	43.4
Farm	120	12*	10*	69	39	17.9	3.0*	4.5*	38.3	45.4
Region:									
Northeast	682	236	218	249	198	13.9	7.2	11.6	23.0	36.7
North Central	723	303	290	255	165	13.0	7.8	13.0	22.8	28.1
South	1,334	532	512	499	302	20.0	11.4	19.4	37.0	45.1
West	723	302	277	266	155	19.4	11.5	18.2	35.1	46.4

*May be unreliable

Source: *Vital and Health Statistics*, Series 10, No. 115

TABLE 2–8. Death Rate for Gallbladder, United States 1980–1984

DEATH RATE	1980	1981	1982	1983	1984
Number	3,110	2,950	3,120	3,170	3,333
Rate per 100,000	1.4	1.3	1.3	1.4	1.3

Source: *Monthly Vital Statistics Report,* 32,33; numbers 9,12,13; September 1984, December 1984, March 1985

native is the dissolving of cholesterol bile duct stones by a new cholesterol solvent, monooctanoin. The bile acids, chenodeoxycholic acid and ursodeoxycholic acid, can be administered orally to decrease the relative secretion of cholesterol in bile, which causes it to change from supersaturated to unsaturated. Cholesterol stones exposed to the unsaturated bile slowly dissolve. Although they have been used successfully in other countries, these agents have not yet been approved for use in the United States.

Mortality data for persons with gallbladder disease between 1980 and 1984 is summarized in Table 2–8.

Predisposing factors or demographic characteristics of those susceptible to gallstones include obesity, cirrhosis, hemolysis, diabetes, advanced age, female gender, using birth control pills, and being an American Indian. Those who are no longer married, earn less than $5,000 a year and live alone outside standard metropolitan statistical areas also have a higher incidence of gallbladder disease (Table 2–9).

GASTRITIS AND DUODENITIS

As the names indicate, gastritis and duodenitis are inflammatory conditions of the stomach and the duodenum. Symptoms include pain, nausea, vomiting, and systemic electrolytic changes. During episodes of acute gastritis, one may develop moderate fever, anorexia, a coated tongue, persistent vomiting, thirst, prostration, and intense epigastric pain. Mild nausea, anorexia, pain, and distention after a small meal are symptomatic of chronic gastritis.

Possible causes include infection and excessive alcohol consumption. Gastritis may be due to either a deficiency or an excess of hydrochloric acid. Deaths from gastritis and duodenitis in the United States in 1979 are summarized in Table 2–10.

Although mortality seems to be more pronounced in men, gastritis and duodenitis patients tend to be older women (Table 2–11, pp. 44–45).

Treatment for chronic gastritis consists of antispasmodics, antacids, sedatives, and avoiding symptom-producing foods. A connection between this condition and specific foods, however, is not currently supported in medical opinion.

DIVERTICULA OF THE INTESTINE

Diverticula are herniations (protrusions) of the colonic mucosa through the bowel wall. They are caused by pressure within the colonic lumen caused by specific foods or emotional stress, muscular thickening, or luminal narrowing. Most diverticula develop in the sigmoid colon.

The most common symptoms are pain, diverticulitis, hemorrhage, obstruction, and—to a lesser extent—fistula formation. Diverticulitis involves abscess and fistula formation and sometimes obstruction. The physician needs to be alert to clinical signs of fever, localized inflammation indicated by left lower abdominal tenderness, and diverticula. The colon shows a saw-toothed appearance on x-ray film.

This condition is rare in Africa, Asia, and Western countries in people younger than age 45 years. This observation, as mentioned in the discussion on constipation, has led to speculation about and research on the possible benefits of a high-fiber diet of 30–37 gms per day. Of older people in industrialized countries, 40% to 45% show signs of this disorder by age 70 years. The reported survey prevalence rate is 31.0 per 1,000 for people older than age 65 years. The number of deaths due to diverticula of the intestine in 1979 according to sex, race, and age is summarized in Table 2–12. The profile of those who exhibit the greatest prevalence of this disease is shown in Table 2–13, pp. 46–47. Nasogastric suction is used for patients with uncomplicated diverticulitis, together with antibiotics. Complicated episodes are treated surgically.

ENTERITIS AND COLITIS

Both these conditions involve inflammation of the colon. Ulcerative colitis usually causes weight loss, lower abdominal pain, and diarrhea, which may be bloody. Stools may be small and frequent, and the colon spasmodic. The sufferer may develop a fever and abdominal distention and tenderness. The rectal mucosa has the texture of sandpaper, is irritable, and bleeds easily.

TABLE 2–9. Number and Rate per 1,000 Population of Gallbladder Conditions Reported in Health Interviews, by Age and Selected Characteristics: United States, 1975 (data are based on household interviews of the civilian noninstitutionalized population)

CHARACTERISTIC	ALL AGES	UNDER 45 YEARS		45–64 YEARS	65 YEARS AND OVER	ALL AGES	UNDER 45 YEARS		45–64 YEARS	65 YEARS AND OVER
		Total	17–44 Years				Total	17–44 Years		
	Number of conditions in thousands					Rate per 1,000 population				
Total	1,625	498	484	659	469	7.8	3.4	5.8	15.3	22.0
Sex:										
Male	304	74	72	137	93	3.0	1.0	1.8	6.7	10.6
Female	1,322	424	411	522	376	12.2	5.8	9.6	23.1	30.1
Race:										
White	1,459	424	414	607	428	8.0	3.4	5.8	15.7	22.1
All other	167	74	70	52	41	6.1	3.6	6.5	11.7	21.0
Black	148	61	57	51	36	6.1	3.3	6.1	12.7	19.7
Usual Activity Status:										
School age (6–16 years)	10*	10*	...	...	...	0.2*	0.2*	...	...	...
Usually working (17 years and over)	504	211	211	254	39	6.3	4.2	4.2	9.4	15.8
Usually keeping house (female, 17 years and over)	895	251	249	337	307	22.3	14.2	14.1	27.8	29.8
Retired (45 years and over)	118	...	...	32*	85	12.0	...	...	13.6*	11.4
Other activity (17 years and over)	92	22*	22*	35	35	5.3	1.5*	1.5*	23.7	33.5
Marital Status:										
Married	1,080	370	370	498	212	11.0	7.1	7.1	14.5	18.4
Formerly married	454	76	76	136	242	21.5	12.2	12.2	21.2	28.6
Widowed	312	4*	4*	80	228	27.1	8.2*	8.2*	23.7	29.7
Separated	51	34*	34*	14*	3*	15.5	16.0*	16.0*	15.2*	12.3*
Divorced	92	38	38	42	11*	14.6	10.5	10.5	20.0	19.8*
Never married	77	38	38	25*	14*	2.7	1.5	1.5	10.9*	10.8*

Employment Status:									
In the labor force (17 years and over)	603	284	284	277	42	6.6	4.7	4.7	9.8	14.0
Employed	554	242	242	264	38	6.5	4.5	4.5	9.9	13.6
Unemployed	59	42	42	13*	4*	7.5	6.9	6.9	8.0*	19.0*
Not in the labor force (17 years and over)	1,009	200	200	382	427	18.0	8.7	8.7	25.9	23.4
Living Arrangements:									
Living alone	265	12*	12*	85	168	17.3	2.2*	2.3*	20.4	28.8
Living with nonrelatives	23*	11*	11*	7*	5*	6.3*	3.9*	3.9*	14.3*	15.9*
Living with spouse	1,070	365	365	496	209	11.0	7.1	7.1	14.5	18.4
Living with other relatives	267	110	96	71	86	2.9	1.3	4.1	16.6	22.9
Family Income:									
Less than $5,000	464	93	87	138	233	14.6	5.1	8.5	26.0	27.9
$5,000–$9,999	399	119	116	180	101	8.8	3.9	6.8	20.6	17.1
$10,000–$14,999	338	144	142	153	41	7.2	4.0	7.0	16.7	19.2
$15,000 or more	313	122	120	147	44	4.5	2.4	4.0	9.3	17.9
Education of Head of Family:									
Less than 12 years	893	201	192	358	335	11.7	4.5	8.3	19.0	25.4
12 years	457	194	190	188	75	6.7	3.8	6.5	14.5	18.6
13–15 years	123	52	52	52	19*	4.3	2.3	3.7	11.2	11.2*
16 years or more	123	48	46	47	28*	3.7	1.9	3.0	8.1	15.1*
Place of Residence:									
SMSA	937	303	299	382	252	6.5	3.0	5.1	12.9	18.7
Central city	414	128	125	172	114	6.7	3.1	5.1	13.3	17.1
Outside central city	523	175	173	210	138	6.4	3.0	5.2	12.5	20.2
Outside SMSA	688	195	185	276	217	10.5	4.4	7.6	20.6	27.8
Nonfarm	602	178	168	232	192	10.3	4.4	7.5	20.0	27.7
Farm	87	17*	17*	44	25*	13.0	4.2*	7.7*	24.4	29.1*
Region:									
Northeast	341	111	109	148	82	6.9	3.4	5.8	13.6	15.2
North Central	500	163	159	189	148	8.9	4.2	7.1	16.9	25.2
South	511	141	134	218	151	7.6	3.0	5.1	16.2	22.6
West	274	83	82	103	88	7.4	3.2	5.4	13.6	26.3

*May be unreliable
Source: *Vital and Health Statistics*, Series 10, No. 115

TABLE 2–10. Mortality Data for Gastritis and Duodenitis, United States, 1979

CHARACTERISTIC	DEATHS
All	648
Male	398
Female	250
White male	342
White female	228
Black male	46
Black female	31
Under age 5 years	2
Age 5–35 years	23
Age 35–50 years	73
Age 50–65 years	168
Age 65+	390

Source: *Vital Statistics, United States, Part II,* 1979

Enteritis and Crohn's disease also cause diarrhea and right lower quadrant pain. A right lower quadrant mass is sometimes palpated on clinical examination. Intestinal obstruction can be a common complication. Diagnosis is made by proctosigmoidoscopy, barium enema, and contrast radiography.

The cause of these inflammatory intestinal diseases is unknown. But several avenues are being explored. The pattern of greater prevalence in certain families suggests a genetic or hereditary component. Patients with inflammatory bowel disease related to ankylosing spondylitis have increased frequency of HLA-B27 antigens, as do other ankylosing spondylitis patients, but no direct connection has been found between HLA-B27 and these bowel disorders. An infection theory has also been explored but no infectious agent found. Researchers are considering a possible altered immune response in patients with Crohn's disease. They have greater levels overall of T-suppressor cells but a lower-than-normal level at the inflammation site. The failure of T-suppressor cells to operate at inflammation sites may cause hypersensitivity to ordinary intestinal antigens that typically do not elicit an immune response. The immunoregulatory role of cells in lesions is currently under intense investigation.

The possibility of prostaglandin treatment to induce greater protection of intestinal mucosa from irritation and inflammation is also being investigated much in the way oral administration of several prostaglandins are being studied with respect to stomach mucosa and ulcers.

Deaths from noninfective gastroenteritis and colitis in 1979 by sex, race, and age are shown in Table 2–14.

It is commonly thought that adults between age 20 and 40 years develop these diseases most often. But government survey data show a pattern of older age incidence that is similar to that of other digestive diseases. Women and whites also seem more susceptible to these diseases (Table 2–15).

No definitive treatment yet exists for these two colonic conditions. Still, steroids and sulfasalazine are used effectively in many patients, especially those with colitis. Unresponsive patients are surgically treated. Operative procedure can be totally effective in treating colitis. This is not the case for Crohn's disease; it can recur after total colectomy.

TABLE 2–12. Mortality Data for Diverticula of the Intestine, United States, 1979

CHARACTERISTICS	NUMBER OF DEATHS
All	2,924
Males	937
Females	1,987
White male	872
White female	1,832
Black male	61
Black female	148
Under age 5 years	1
Age 5–35 years	4
Age 35–50 years	47
Age 50–65 years	373
Age 65+	2,923

Source: *Vital Statistics, United States, Part II* 1979

TABLE 2–14. Mortality Data for Noninfective Gastroenteritis and Colitis in 1979

CHARACTERISTICS	NUMBER OF DEATHS
All	5,719
Male	2,363
Female	3,356
White Male	2,070
White Female	3,054
Black Male*	257
Black Female*	278
Under Age 5	277
Age 5–35	76
Age 35–50	169
Age 50–65	836
Age 65+	4,356

Source: *Vital Statistics, United States, Part II,* 1979
*Does not include non-white

TABLE 2–11. Number and Rate per 1,000 Population of Gastritis and Duodenitis Reported in Health Interviews, by Age and Selected Characteristics: United States, 1975 (data are based on household interviews of the civilian noninstitutionalized population)

CHARACTERISTICS	ALL AGES	UNDER 45 YEARS Total	UNDER 45 YEARS 17–44 Years	45–64 YEARS	65 YEARS AND OVER	ALL AGES	UNDER 45 YEARS Total	UNDER 45 YEARS 17–44 Years	45–64 YEARS	65 YEARS AND OVER
	Number of conditions in thousands					Rate per 1,000 population				
Total	1,465	604	533	431	370	70	4.2	6.4	11.4	17.4
Sex:										
Male	588	272	236	181	135	5.8	3.8	5.9	8.8	15.4
Female	878	332	297	311	235	8.1	4.5	6.9	13.8	18.8
Race:										
White	1,278	509	441	435	334	7.0	4.1	6.1	11.2	17.3
All other	188	96	92	56	36	6.9	4.6	8.6	12.6	18.5
Black	177	89	85	52	36	7.3	4.8	9.1	13.0	19.7
Usual Activity Status:										
School age (6–16 years)	46	46	...	...	...	1.1	1.1	...	...	...
Usually working (17 years and over)	579	315	315	221	44	7.3	6.3	6.3	8.2	17.8
Usually keeping house (female, 17 years and over)	540	144	144	204	192	13.4	8.1	8.1	16.8	18.6
Retired (45 years and over)	141	...	...	39	102	14.4	...	...	16.6	13.7
Other activity (17 years and over)	135	75	75	28*	32*	7.7	5.0	5.0	18.9*	30.6*
Marital Status:										
Married	898	353	353	344	201	9.2	6.8	6.8	10.0	17.4
Formerly married	327	78	78	108	141	15.5	12.5	12.5	16.9	16.6
Widowed	182	5*	5*	57	119	15.8	10.3*	10.3*	16.9	15.5
Separated	42	25*	25*	12*	5*	12.8	11.7*	11.7*	13.0*	20.6*
Divorced	103	47	47	39	17*	16.4	13.0	13.0	18.5	30.6*
Never married	170	103	103	39	27*	6.0	4.2	4.2	17.0	20.8*

Employment Status:										
In the labor force (17 years and over)	646	360	360	236	50	7.1	6.0	6.0	8.3	16.6
Employed	582	320	320	215	46	7.0	6.0	6.0	8.1	16.4
Unemployed	64	40	40	21*	3*	8.1	6.6	6.6	13.0*	14.3*
Not in the labor force (17 years and over)	749	173	173	255	320	13.4	7.5	7.5	17.3	17.5
Living Arrangements:										
Living alone	257	51	51	86	121	16.8	9.5	9.6	20.6	20.8
Living with nonrelatives	31*	18*	18*	7*	5*	8.5*	6.3*	6.4*	14.3*	15.9*
Living with spouse	889	350	350	342	196	9.2	6.8	6.8	10.0	17.2
Living with other relatives	289	185	114	56	47	3.1	2.2	4.9	13.1	12.5
Family Income:										
Less than $5,000	366	67	60	133	167	11.5	3.7	5.9	25.0	20.0
$5,000–$9,999	339	136	126	104	99	7.5	4.4	7.4	11.9	16.7
$10,000–$14,999	308	164	140	106	38	6.5	4.6	6.9	11.5	17.8
$15,000 or more	377	225	197	119	33*	5.4	4.4	6.5	7.5	13.5*
Education of Head of Family:										
Less than 12 years	669	159	137	243	268	8.7	3.6	5.9	12.9	20.3
12 years	420	216	189	152	52	6.2	4.2	6.4	11.7	12.9
13–15 years	166	113	109	41	12*	5.8	5.1	7.8	8.8	7.1*
16 years or more	200	117	98	47	36	6.1	4.7	6.4	8.1	19.4
Place of Residence:										
SMSA	1,032	460	418	337	235	7.2	4.6	7.2	11.3	17.4
Central city	522	217	200	178	127	8.5	5.2	8.1	13.8	19.0
Outside central city	510	244	218	159	108	6.2	4.2	6.5	9.5	15.8
Outside SMSA	433	144	116	155	134	6.6	3.3	4.7	11.6	17.2
Nonfarm	398	132	112	146	120	6.8	3.3	5.0	12.6	17.3
Farm	35	12*	4*	9*	14*	5.2	3.0*	1.8*	5.0*	16.3*
Region:										
Northeast	363	139	115	124	100	7.4	4.2	6.1	11.4	18.5
North Central	391	164	156	127	100	7.0	4.2	7.0	11.4	17.1
South	366	149	131	125	91	5.5	3.2	5.0	9.3	13.6
West	346	152	131	115	79	9.3	5.8	8.6	15.2	23.6

*May be unreliable
Source: *Vital and Health Statistics*, Series 10, No. 115

TABLE 2–13. Number and Rate per 1,000 Population of Diverticula of Intestine Reported in Health Interviews, by Age and Selected Characteristics: United States, 1975 (data are based on household interviews of the civilian noninstitutionalized population)

CHARACTERISTIC	Number of conditions in thousands					Rate per 1,000 population				
	ALL AGES	UNDER 45 YEARS Total	UNDER 45 YEARS 17–44 Years	45–64 YEARS	65 YEARS AND OVER	ALL AGES	UNDER 45 YEARS Total	UNDER 45 YEARS 17–44 Years	45–64 YEARS	65 YEARS AND OVER
Total	1,323	94	94	569	660	6.3	0.6	1.1	13.2	31.0
Sex:										
Male	366	23*	23*	190	153	3.6	0.3*	0.6*	9.3	17.4
Female	957	71	71	379	507	8.8	1.0	1.7	16.8	40.5
Race:										
White	1,305	94	94	561	654	7.2	0.8	1.3	14.5	33.8
All other	18*	4*	4*	8*	6*	0.7*	0.2*	0.4*	1.8*	3.1*
Black	18*	4*	4*	8*	6*	0.7*	0.2*	0.4*	2.0*	3.3*
Usual Activity Status:										
School age (6–16 years)	...	...	...	...	...	...	...	...	...	...
Usually working (17 years and over)	379	56	56	283	40	4.8	1.1	1.1	10.5	16.2
Usually keeping house (female, 17 years and over)	571	29*	29*	225	417	16.7	1.6	1.6	18.5	40.5
Retired (45 years and over)	195	...	...	42	154	19.9	...	...	17.8	20.7
Other activity (17 years and over)	76	9*	9*	18*	49	4.4	0.6	0.6*	12.2*	46.9
Marital Status:										
Married	859	70	70	439	349	8.8	1.3	1.3	12.8	30.3
Formerly married	378	12*	12*	94	272	17.9	1.9*	1.9*	14.7	32.1
Widowed	319	2*	2*	61	256	27.7	4.1*	4.1*	18.1	33.4
Separated	14*	3*	3*	9*	2*	4.3*	1.4*	1.4*	9.8*	8.2*
Divorced	45	7*	7*	24*	14*	7.2	1.9*	1.9*	11.4*	25.2*
Never married	87	12*	12*	36	38	3.1	0.5*	0.5*	15.7	29.3

Employment Status:										
In the labor force (17 years and over)	424	64	64	300	60	4.7	1.1	1.1	10.6	19.9
Employed	405	63	63	284	58	4.9	1.2	1.2	10.6	20.7
Unemployed	19*	2*	2*	16*	2*	2.4*	0.3*	0.3*	9.9*	9.5*
Not in the labor force (17 years and over)	899	30*	30*	270	600	16.1	1.3*	1.3*	18.3	32.8
Living Arrangements:										
Living alone	304	2*	2*	87	216	19.8	0.4*	0.4*	20.9	37.1
Living with nonrelatives	22*	2*	2*	13*	7*	6.0*	0.7*	0.7*	26.5*	22.2*
Living with spouse	850	70	70	438	343	8.8	1.4	1.4	12.8	30.1
Living with other relatives	147	21*	21*	32*	94	1.6	0.2*	0.9*	7.5*	25.0
Family Income:										
Less than $5,000	290	5*	5*	75	211	9.1	0.3*	0.5*	14.1	25.2
$5,000–$9,999	341	17*	17*	124	200	7.5	0.6*	1.0*	14.2	33.8
$10,000–$14,999	225	23*	23*	121	81	4.8	0.6*	1.1*	13.2	37.9
$15,000 or more	338	44	44	208	86	4.8	0.9	1.5	13.2	35.1
Education of Head of Family:										
Less than 12 years	519	15*	15*	193	311	6.8	0.3*	0.6*	10.2	23.5
12 years	375	34*	34*	190	151	5.5	0.7*	1.2*	14.6	37.4
13–15 years	203	28*	28*	81	94	7.1	1.3*	2.0*	17.4	55.5
16 years or more	210	18*	18*	98	95	6.4	0.7*	1.2*	16.9	51.3
Place of Residence:										
SMSA	919	84	84	409	426	6.4	0.8	1.4	13.8	31.6
Central city	360	19*	19*	176	165	5.8	0.5*	0.8*	13.6	24.7
Outside central city	559	65	65	233	261	6.8	1.1	1.9	13.9	38.3
Outside SMSA	404	10*	10*	161	233	6.2	0.2*	0.4*	12.0	29.9
Nonfarm	367	10*	10*	143	214	6.3	0.2*	0.4*	12.4	30.9
Farm	37	...	...	18*	20*	5.5	...	...	10.0*	23.3*
Region:										
Northeast	360	30*	30*	151	179	7.3	0.9*	1.6*	13.9	33.2
North Central	307	19*	19*	142	146	5.5	0.5*	0.9*	12.7	24.9
South	372	26*	26*	137	209	5.6	0.6*	1.0*	10.2	31.2
West	284	19*	19*	139	126	7.6	0.7*	1.2*	18.3	37.7

*May be unreliable
Source: Vital and Health Statistics, Series 10, No. 115

TABLE 2–15. Number and Rate per 1,000 Population of Chronic Enteritis and Colitis Reported in Health Interviews, by Age and Selected Characteristics: United States, 1975 (data are based on household interviews of the civilian noninstitutionalized population)

CHARACTERISTICS	ALL AGES	UNDER 45 YEARS		45–64 YEARS	65 YEARS AND OVER	ALL AGES	UNDER 45 YEARS		45–64 YEARS	65 YEARS AND OVER
		Total	17–44 Years				Total	17–44 Years		
	Number of conditions in thousands					Rate per 1,000 population				
Total	1,183	479	433	416	287	5.7	3.3	5.2	9.7	13.5
Sex:										
Male	361	149	122	137	75	3.6	2.1	3.1	6.7	8.5
Female	822	331	311	279	212	7.6	4.5	7.3	12.4	17.0
Race:										
White	1,145	460	415	403	282	6.3	3.7	5.8	10.4	14.6
All other	38	19*	17*	14*	5*	1.4	0.9*	1.6*	3.2*	2.6*
Black	31*	13*	12*	14*	4*	1.3*	0.7*	1.3*	3.5*	2.2*
Usual Activity Status:										
School age (6–16 years)	18*	18*	…	…	…	0.4*	0.4*	…	…	…
Usually working (17 years and over)	422	227	227	183	12*	5.3	4.5	4.5	6.8	4.9*
Usually keeping house (female, 17 years and over)	507	158	158	176	173	12.6	8.9	8.9	14.5	16.8
Retired (45 years and over)	108	…	…	36	72	11.0	…	…	15.3	9.7
Other activity (17 years and over)	99	48	48	20*	31*	5.7	3.2	3.2	13.5*	29.7*
Marital Status:										
Married	759	321	321	296	141	7.8	6.2	6.2	8.6	12.2
Formerly married	273	43	43	89	141	12.9	6.9	6.9	13.9	16.6
Widowed	175	2*	2*	50	122	15.2	4.1*	4.1*	14.8	15.9
Separated	29*	13*	13*	10*	7*	8.8*	6.1*	6.1*	10.9*	28.8*
Divorced	69	28*	28*	29*	11*	11.0	7.7*	7.7*	13.7*	19.8*
Never married	105	69	69	31*	5*	3.7	2.8	2.8	13.5*	3.9*

Employment Status:										
In the labor force (17 years and over)	486	267	267	203	15*	5.3	4.5	4.5	7.2	5.0*
Employed	432	229	229	189	14*	5.2	4.3	4.3	7.1	5.0*
Unemployed	54	38	38	14*	2*	6.8	6.3	6.3	8.6*	9.5*
Not in the labor force (17 years and over)	651	166	166	214	272	11.6	7.2	7.2	14.5	14.9
Living Arrangements:										
Living alone	216	35	35	79	102	14.1	6.5	6.6	18.9	17.5
Living with nonrelatives	32*	18*	18*	11*	4*	8.7*	6.3*	6.4*	22.4*	12.7
Living with spouse	747	316	316	291	140	7.7	6.2	6.2	8.5	12.3
Living with other relatives	188	110	64	35	42	2.0	1.3	2.8	8.2	11.2
Family Income:										
Less than $5,000	264	63	53	80	122	8.3	3.5	5.2	15.1	14.6
$5,000–$9,999	227	71	66	80	76	5.0	2.3	3.9	9.2	12.8
$10,000–$14,999	216	89	82	91	36	4.6	2.5	4.0	9.9	16.8
$15,000 or more	394	232	210	140	23*	5.6	4.5	7.0	8.9	9.4*
Education of Head of Family										
Less than 12 years	417	74	58	159	184	5.4	1.7	2.5	8.4	13.9
12 years	393	178	169	146	68	5.8	3.5	5.7	11.2	16.9
13–15 years	148	84	74	41	23*	5.2	3.8	5.3	8.8	13.6*
16 years or more	220	141	131	67	12*	6.7	5.6	8.6	11.5	6.5
Place of Residence:										
SMSA	794	359	326	275	160	5.5	3.6	5.6	9.3	11.9
Central city	304	115	101	118	71	4.9	2.7	4.1	9.1	10.6
Outside central city	489	244	225	157	88	6.0	4.2	6.7	9.4	12.9
Outside SMSA	389	120	107	142	128	6.0	2.7	4.4	10.6	16.4
Nonfarm	351	115	102	115	121	6.0	2.9	4.6	9.9	17.4
Farm	38	5*	5*	26*	7*	5.7	1.2*	2.3*	14.4*	8.1*
Region:										
Northeast	281	107	97	103	70	5.7	3.3	5.1	9.5	13.0
North Central	345	151	138	110	84	6.2	3.9	6.2	9.8	14.3
South	313	111	98	129	72	4.7	2.4	3.7	9.6	10.8
West	244	110	99	74	61	6.6	4.2	6.5	9.8	18.2

*May be unreliable

Source: *Vital and Health Statistics*, Series 10, No. 115

Diseases of
3 The Liver

HEPATITIS

Literally, hepatitis means inflammation of the liver. This viral disease has three forms: hepatitis A, commonly called infectious hepatitis; hepatitis B, or serum hepatitis; and non-A, non-B hepatitis. A fourth type, delta hepatitis, is believed to be a parasitic form caused by the recently identified delta agent, which requires the hepatitis B virus to replicate. All three primary forms can have similar symptoms, including fever, loss of appetite, headache, malaise, weakness, muscle pain, and jaundice. Symptoms are typically most acute within 2 weeks after the illness appears and usually subside within 6 weeks. Jaundice, or yellowing of the skin, is often accompanied by nausea, vomiting, abdominal discomfort, mental depression, and irritability. The liver becomes large and tender. Acute infections are in the main nonicteric (not jaundice-producing).

The mildest form of hepatitis is infectious type A, although both types A and B can be acute or almost nonsymptomatic. Type A is spread primarily in contaminated drinking water or food. But an infected person incubating the hepatitis A virus can spread the infection to close contacts, especially during the 7 days before symptoms develop. Often, contacts are given immunoglobulin to help them resist infection. This procedure is recommended mainly for close family members but generally not for school or work contacts.

Type B hepatitis is a viral disease spread through blood products and other bodily fluids, such as saliva and semen. Typically, hepatitis B lasts no longer than 6 months unless it becomes chronic. Type B usually causes both more severe illness than type A and more fatalities, as well as a greater incidence of ensuing chronic hepatic disease. Some patients with type B have the chronic form and can transmit it to others through bodily fluids.

The third form of the disease was identified in 1975. It seems to be caused by several viral agents but not by the ones that cause types A and B. So, instead of referring to this third type as type C, it is simply called non-A, non-B hepatitis. It is most often transmitted by blood transfusion and is diagnosed by ruling out types A and B. The profile of non-A, non-B hepatitis closely resembles type B. Either of these diseases can lead to chronic hepatitis; type A, however, is not known to lead to chronic liver disease.

Progress in determining the cause and in understanding the course and sequelae of viral hepatitis has been rapid and recent. Just 40 years ago, virtually nothing was known about viral hepatitis. It was confused with several other disorders involving liver dysfunction. The Australian antigen (Au) or HBsAg identified with type B hepatitis was discovered in 1955. This agent was rarely found in healthy populations in the United States. Indeed, it caused a positive test reaction in only 1 of every 1,000 serums tested. But it was common in some tropical and Asian populations. The incidence rate of hepatitis B antigen level in Filipinos from the region of Cebu is estimated at 6%; in the Japanese, 1%; and in certain Pacific island populations, 5% to 15%.

By the 1960s the Au antibody was identified in many transfused patients, especially leukemia patients. It was related not only to the transfusion but also to the leukemia. At first, researchers thought the high transfusion rate of leukemia patients accounted for their higher incidence of hepatitis or for the Au antigen, or both. But they soon hypothesized that leukemia patients showed signs of hepatitis at a rate that was higher than what might be expected in even high-risk transfusion populations. They theorized that the hepatitis virus was related to the leukemia-producing virus.

Other investigators concluded that leukemia is more likely in persons with the Au antigen in their blood than in those without it. Investigators also speculated that persons more likely to develop leukemia, such as children with Down's syndrome, might be more susceptible to the hepatitis antigen as well. Higher-than-average incidences of hepatitis and leukemia have been found in children with Down's syndrome.

By 1966, W. Thomas Landon established that Au antigen was in the blood of many patients in the early stages of hepatitis but then disappeared. Also in 1966, evidence from researchers in Philadelphia confirmed that Au antigen was associated with acute viral hepatitis. Japanese researchers established shortly thereafter that Au antigen associated with hepatitis B could be transmitted by blood transfusion and that acute hepatitis infection followed. By the fall of 1969, all donor blood was tested for the Au antigen; donor blood testing positive was excluded from banks. This reduced the incidence of posttransfusion hepatitis to 6%. This one discovery and prevention measure saves the United States one-half-billion dollars of health-resource expenditures annually.

INCIDENCE

Scientists at the National Institutes of Health (NIH) estimate that as many as 500,000 cases of hepatitis occur annually in the United States. The number actually reported is considerably lower, however. Several individual epidemiologic studies indicate that the under-reporting rate for type A hepatitis is as high as 70%. This type of hepatitis usually invites more public-health attention because of its spread through food and water. Conceivably, therefore, type B hepatitis, which is transmitted on a more individual basis, is equally under-reported.

The Centers for Disease Control (CDC) Program in Atlanta, Georgia, receives reports from states and U.S. territories and disseminates information about the disease and patient in *Morbidity and Mortality Weekly Reports* (MMWR). Another network is the Viral Hepatitis Surveillance Program, a voluntary state reporting system operated by the Division of Hepatitis and Viral Enteritis Center for Infectious Disease (HVEC), part of the CDC. This reporting system includes more epidemiologic information than the Atlanta *MMWR* program, but HVEC lists fewer cases because all their reports are voluntary. In 1981, the HVEC system reported only 47% of the cases reported to the Atlanta program.

In 1983, a total of 56,469 cases of viral hepatitis was reported to the National Morbidity Reporting System. This figure represented an incidence rate of 24.1 per 100,000 for the United States. Thirty-eight percent of the reported cases were hepatitis A; 43% were hepatitis B, and 6.1% were non-A, non-B. More than 7,000 cases remained unspecified. The overall incidence of hepatitis reported between 1975 and 1983 has been decreasing, although there were marked changes for the specific types of hepatitis. Hepatitis B exceeded hepatitis A for the first time in 1983 (Fig. 3–1).

FIG. 3–1.   Hepatitis: reported cases per 100,000 population, by year, United States, 1955–1983

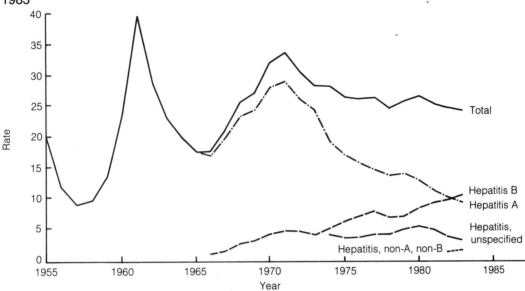

Source: *National Surveillance Viral Hepatitis Program*, 1983

Reported cases of each type of viral hepatitis vary according to locale (Figs. 3–2 and 3–3). The highest rates of reported hepatitis A came from Texas and other western and southwestern states; the highest incidence of hepatitis B was reported in the east and west coast states. Reporting of non-A, non-B is so new that the data are not yet considered to be reliable.

The number of hepatitis A cases reported by each state in 1981 according to age is summarized in Table 3–1.

Hepatitis B cases reported according to age in each case are presented in Table 3–2.

Unspecified cases not identified as type A, type B or non-A, non-B reported by state in 1981 according to age are presented in Table 3–3.

Certain major demographic characteristics are associated with the three kinds of hepatitis perhaps more markedly than with most other diseases.

These age, race, and sex characteristics are presented in Table 3–4.

Another characteristic most often associated with hepatitis A patients is contact with people who have hepatitis A or who have had contact with a child or day-care center. Hepatitis B sufferers are

FIG. 3–2.   Hepatitis A: reported cases of hepatitis A per 100,000 population, by state, United States, 1983

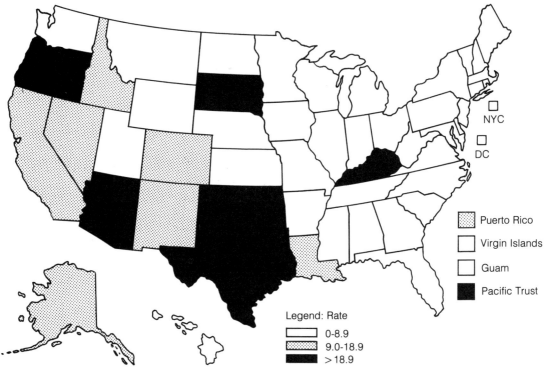

Source: *National Surveillance of Viral Hepatitis,* 1983

often health-care workers, comprising as much as 18% of type B patients in some states. Some patients are also active homosexuals. They account for up to 21% of the cases in various states. Substantial numbers of hepatitis B and of non-A, non-B hepatitis patients were hospitalized just before their illness (Table 3–5). Epidemiologists suspect hepatitis was transmitted to them through blood transfusion and that this accounts for the many people older than age 60 years with non-A, non-B hepatitis. In some states, as many as 20% of non-A, non-B hepatitis patients reported being I.V. drug users. Another 16% reported being employed in the medical or dental fields, or both, in some states although an average incidence of only 7% was reported across the country.

Hepatitis is endemic in large portions of the world. An estimated 200 million people are chronically infected with hepatitis B virus, which often leads to cirrhosis of the liver and liver cancer. People

FIG. 3–3.   Hepatitis B

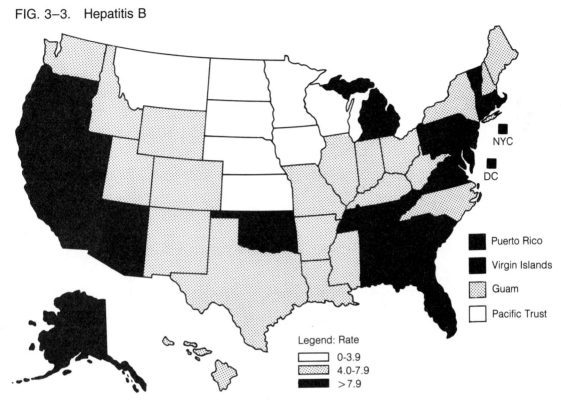

Source: *National Surveillance of Viral Hepatitis,* 1983.

in southeast Asia, the Pacific islands and sub-Saharan Africa have more than a 50% lifetime risk of acquiring a hepatitis B virus (HBV) infection. Most infections occur perinatally when infants are directly infected by their mother or during childhood. In the regions just cited, few people develop acute hepatitis with jaundice, but 5% to 20% become chronic viral carriers and die from cirrhosis or primary hepatocellular carcinoma (PHC). Chronic HBV infection in which the patient is in the chronic HBsAg carrier state is the major cause of cirrhosis worldwide. Of those who develop liver cancer where the chronic HBsAg carrier state is endemic, 70% to 90% are chronically infected with hepatitis B. The risk of hepatic cancer is 300- to 400-fold among those who become infected at birth. Liver cancer is one of the most common causes of death in these regions. Even in the United States, 6,000 new cases are reported annually.

In North America and western Europe, the lifetime risk of hep-

TABLE 3–1. Hepatitis A: Reported Cases, by Area and Age, United States, 1981

AREA	TOTAL ALL AGES	UNDER 1	1–4	5–9	10–14	15–19	20–24	25–29	30–39	40–49	50–59	60+	UN-KNOWN
United States	25,802	57	848	2,181	1,828	2,731	4,976	4,209	4,108	1,528*	1,151*	1,271*	790
New England	699	—	7	10	33	85	151	126	116	55	43	47	26
Maine	39	—	—	—	3	—	6	3	6	4	2	6	9
N.H.	56	—	3	1	—	4	5	10	13	3	3	7	7
Vt.	50	—	1	1	5	7	8	6	8	6	4	4	—
Mass.	265	—	—	6	14	36	54	59	45	17	13	15	6
R.I.	99	—	1	—	5	16	22	17	17	9	7	5	—
Conn.	190	—	2	2	6	22	56	31	27	16	14	10	4
Mid. Atlantic	3,157	3	32	112	159	355	662	493	575	271	239	227	29
N.Y. (excl. NYC)	645	—	14	45	41	68	91	78	122	48	62	64	12
N.Y.C.	606†	1	3	19	33	44	109	122	117	53	45	57	3
N.J.	1,124	2	6	16	47	144	272	159	202	109	90	63	14
Pa.	782	—	9	32	38	99	190	134	134	61	42	43	—
E.N. Central	3,286	15	138	338	293	356	527	469	470	145*	119*	157*	135
Ohio	699	4	29	42	57	79	134	97	92	32	34	50	49
Ind.	684	2	41	118	88	73	104	90	71	36	29	21	11
Ill.	864	2	40	114	97	91	128	108	129	———	124	———	31
Mich.	794	3	16	51	46	92	107	131	139	69	46	70	24
Wis.	245	4	12	13	5	21	54	43	39	8	10	16	20
W.N. Central	884	2	19	78	53	86	148	148	141	53	52	70	34
Minn.	116	—	1	6	6	7	20	21	26	4	12	13	—
Iowa	217	1	7	33	15	28	26	35	28	10	12	15	7
Mo.	282	1	4	14	18	25	55	53	52	16	15	15	14
N. Dak.	14	—	—	1	—	2	4	—	2	1	1	3	—
S. Dak.	38	—	2	2	6	5	5	2	4	1	3	6	2
Nebr.	46	—	—	4	5	4	6	7	8	5	3	3	1
Kans.	171	—	5	18	3	15	32	30	21	16	6	15	10
S. Atlantic	3,055	10	87	157	130	288	635	515	530	195	178	247	83
Del.	73	—	1	2	—	14	20	18	5	—	2	3	8
Md.	211	—	4	7	8	19	49	44	26	22	17	15	—
D.C.	44	—	1	1	—	—	8	4	13	3	6	1	7
Va.	200	—	3	2	3	18	36	37	36	18	17	25	5

Area												
W. Va.	109	1	1	4	4	11	18	18	16	8	7	14	7
N.C.	252	—	3	4	10	24	45	39	43	21	26	34	3
S.C.	114	—	1	2	2	17	23	17	18	5	7	17	5
Ga.	543	4	14	21	22	35	113	84	93	35	36	47	39
Fla.	1,509	5	59	114	81	150	323	254	280	83	61	91	9
E.S. Central	1,183	5	33	114	113	146	212	163	147	77	16	95	17
Ky.	345	1	15	54	41	35	50	39	45	22	20	21	6
Tenn.	435	2	7	36	46	56	85	67	56	30	10	30	—
Ala.	153	—	1	5	11	23	40	19	18	10	10	15	1
Miss.	250	2	10	19	15	32	37	38	28	15	15	29	10
W.S. Central	4,060	6	210	625	471	467	670	541	519	162	102	145	142
Ark.	243	1	6	18	16	23	49	39	44	15	7	19	6
La.	772	1	42	64	67	93	127	128	117	32	26	23	52
Okla.	324	—	17	49	28	45	54	36	36	18	11	14	16
Tex.	2,721	4	145	494	360	306	440	338	322	97	58	89	68
Mountain	2,090	8	126	242	166	162	407	305	345	114	77	46	92
Mont.	98	—	5	11	7	4	18	16	17	6	4	7	3
Idaho	265	—	15	44	23	24	36	33	41	11	10	4	24
Wyo.	77	—	3	7	7	6	16	6	19	3	2	3	5
Colo.	561	—	22	41	36	34	120	111	116	40	16	8	17
N. Mex.	281	2	21	46	31	31	51	33	31	10	16	2	7
Ariz.	503	6	50	75	42	41	107	53	66	18	16	16	13
Utah	104	—	4	8	7	8	15	17	23	13	4	3	2
Nev.	201	—	6	10	13	14	44	36	32	13	9	3	21
Pacific	7,388	8	196	505	410	786	1,564	1,449	1,265	456	280	237	232
Wash.	791	2	33	66	68	70	132	133	139	59	37	29	23
Oreg.	518	1	11	25	22	33	95	129	105	38	26	25	8
Calif.	5,910	5	151	414	317	665	1,275	1,151	992	351	213	178	198
Alaska	45	—	1	1	2	4	10	14	9	6	2	1	1
Hawaii	124	—	—	—	1	14	52	22	20	13	2	2	2
Guam	14	—	—	—	—	1	5	4	—	—	4	2	2
P.R.	370	2	11	66	46	65	66	41	38	13	1	9	9
V.I.	4	—	—	—	—	—	1	1	—	—	—	—	1
Pac. Trust Terr.	15	—	—	—	—	—	NA	—	—	—	—	—	15
C.N.M.I.	—	—	—	—	—	—	—	—	—	—	—	—	—

*Does not include cases reported by state of Illinois
†Cases represent patients tested for HBsAg and found to be negative
Source: *Atlanta Center For Disease Control*

TABLE 3–2.　Hepatitis B: Reported Cases, by Area and Age, United States, 1981

AREA	TOTAL ALL AGES	UNDER 1	1–4	5–9	10–14	15–19	20–24	25–29	30–39	40–49	50–59	60+	UN-KNOWN
United States	21,152	49	80	113	168	2,391	5,530	4,184	3,702	1,533*	1,112*	1,305*	722
New England	1,090	2	—	4	3	101	322	232	161	79	68	74	44
Maine	42	—	—	1	—	4	4	4	8	5	—	3	13
N.H.	43	—	—	—	—	4	15	10	6	2	2	1	3
Vt.	28	—	—	—	—	1	9	1	7	3	3	4	—
Mass.	374	1	—	1	2	42	102	82	57	31	16	26	14
R.I.	87	—	—	—	—	5	30	19	16	7	4	6	—
Conn.	516	1	—	2	1	45	162	116	67	31	43	34	14
Mid. Atlantic	3,740	7	14	16	29	406	1,024	731	699	267	229	275	43
N.Y. (excl. NYC)	719†	2	2	2	10	64	178	126	125	64	52	67	27
N.Y.C.	879	1	4	5	8	91	208	166	200	67	57	66	6
N.J.	1,198	4	5	4	6	144	385	243	188	78	64	67	10
Pa.	944	—	3	5	5	107	253	196	186	58	56	75	—
E.N. Central	2,696	10	9	11	25	288	668	538	465	149*	104*	135*	91
Ohio	719	1	4	3	6	94	194	144	101	54	39	49	30
Ind.	413	—	1	—	5	53	128	81	59	28	22	25	11
Ill.	711	5	—	3	6	49	141	134	151	203 (40–49 & 50–59 combined)		—	19
Mich.	687	3	4	5	4	65	173	144	128	57	35	51	18
Wis.	166	1	—	—	4	27	32	35	26	10	8	10	13
W.N. Central	705	—	1	1	7	78	152	146	125	70	43	39	43
Minn.	134	—	—	—	—	10	34	27	30	19	11	2	1
Iowa	94	—	1	1	—	15	15	20	12	14	8	6	2
Mo.	307	—	—	—	5	32	59	59	57	25	20	18	32
N. Dak.	5	—	—	—	1	1	—	—	—	2	—	1	—
S. Dak.	8	—	—	—	—	1	3	1	2	—	1	—	—
Nebr.	75	—	—	—	1	10	19	21	13	4	2	4	1
Kans.	82	—	—	—	—	9	22	18	11	6	1	8	7
S. Atlantic	4,744	10	14	19	28	496	1,196	936	875	379	264	339	188
Del.	95	—	—	1	1	6	22	14	12	7	5	1	26
Md.	759	2	1	2	5	98	251	169	130	38	31	31	1
D.C.	110	—	—	—	—	7	24	14	31	9	2	6	17
Va.	537	—	2	2	3	57	134	105	102	42	33	37	20
W. Va.	122	—	—	—	1	15	24	20	22	7	14	13	6

N.C.	347	—	1	—	1	34	80	70	70	32	27	28	4
S.C.	446	2	1	3	4	54	111	93	79	38	22	23	16
Ga.	816	2	5	5	9	78	158	149	160	71	48	56	75
Fla.	1,512	4	4	6	4	147	392	302	269	135	82	144	23
E.S. Central	1,107	3	3	7	7	150	280	223	162	98	65	105	4
Ky.	173	—	—	—	—	25	45	35	22	20	9	15	2
Tenn.	518	2	1	1	3	55	117	97	87	48	41	65	1
Ala.	288	1	2	5	3	41	84	69	43	19	10	11	—
Miss.	128	—	—	1	1	29	34	22	10	11	5	14	1
W.S. Central	1,541	6	13	16	21	184	368	302	249	122	78	109	73
Ark.	99	—	—	1	2	12	20	14	15	7	3	14	11
La.	363	2	2	1	5	43	101	70	41	29	20	20	31
Okla.	256	2	2	2	6	33	53	54	55	16	9	14	10
Tex.	823	4	9	12	8	96	194	164	138	70	46	61	21
Mountain	782	2	4	6	10	76	161	152	148	65	42	39	77
Mont.	25	—	—	1	1	2	6	2	5	2	—	2	4
Idaho	21	—	—	—	2	6	2	2	2	1	1	1	5
Wyo.	16	—	—	—	—	1	3	5	3	2	—	1	—
Colo.	220	—	3	1	3	20	54	45	49	17	9	7	12
N. Mex.	77	—	—	1	—	6	18	16	16	6	3	7	4
Ariz.	191	2	1	1	2	14	41	40	41	23	11	15	2
Utah	55	—	—	1	2	8	10	10	9	4	7	1	3
Nev.	177	—	—	1	2	19	27	32	23	10	11	5	47
Pacific	4,747	9	22	33	38	612	1,359	924	878	304	219	190	159
Wash.	345	3	3	5	2	32	93	69	69	27	11	13	18
Oreg.	358	1	5	1	4	31	77	84	80	28	14	15	18
Calif.	3,876	12	12	23	32	540	1,150	744	692	236	182	146	118
Alaska	73	3	2	3	—	1	12	10	18	10	7	6	3
Hawaii	95	1	—	1	—	8	27	17	21	3	5	10	2
Guam	7	—	—	—	—	1	1	1	2	1	—	1	—
P.R.	169	2	1	6	7	29	48	34	19	5	2	8	8
V.I.	2	—	—	—	—	—	—	2	—	—	—	—	—
Pac. Trust Terr.	—	—	—	—	—	—	—	—	—	—	—	—	—
C.N.M.I.	—	—	—	—	—	—	—	—	—	—	—	—	—

*Does not include cases reported by state of Illinois
†Cases represent patients tested for HBsAg and found to be positive
Source: *Atlanta Centers For Disease Control*

TABLE 3–3. Hepatitis, Unspecified: Reported Cases, by Area and Age, United States, 1981

AREA	TOTAL ALL AGES	UNDER 1	1–4	5–9	10–14	15–19	20–24	25–29	30–39	40–49	50–59	60+	UNKNOWN
United States	10,975	31	276	706	584	1,161	2,230	1,666	1,520	728*	570*	798*	628
New England	311	—	3	4	10	28	60	51	52	27	10	33	33
Maine	15	—	—	—	1	2	1	1	—	1	—	3	6
N.H.	24	—	—	—	3	—	4	1	3	3	—	2	8
Vt.	5	—	—	—	—	—	1	—	3	—	—	1	—
Mass.	197	—	3	3	5	22	45	36	29	16	6	14	18
R.I.	—	—	—	—	—	—	—	—	—	—	—	—	—
Conn.	70	—	—	1	1	4	9	13	17	7	4	13	1
Mid. Atlantic	1,244	1	11	27	49	142	286	194	188	98	105	128	15
N.Y. (excl. NYC)	251	—	6	10	15	15	50	33	30	24	25	37	6
N.Y.C.	237†	1	4	17	10	32	54	40	41	12	17	7	2
N.J.	546	—	1	—	16	69	134	94	80	43	50	52	7
Pa.	210	—	—	—	8	26	48	27	37	19	13	32	—
E.N. Central	1,006	5	17	51	37	121	185	148	151	57*	57*	72*	28
Ohio	331	3	6	18	12	38	64	45	60	26	15	31	13
Ind.	244	1	9	14	11	31	52	41	30	12	22	14	7
Ill.	201	1	1	10	6	14	20	35	32	—	77	—	5
Mich.	219	—	1	9	7	36	44	26	29	19	19	26	5
Wis.	11	—	—	—	1	2	5	1	—	—	1	1	3
W.N. Central	393	2	3	21	13	34	69	69	56	37	17	45	27
Minn.	49	—	—	2	1	5	9	10	8	8	3	3	—
Iowa	59	—	—	4	6	4	7	11	7	4	2	10	4
Mo.	214	1	1	10	4	20	40	36	31	18	10	23	20
N. Dak.	5	—	—	—	—	—	—	1	1	1	—	2	—
S. Dak.	2	—	—	—	—	—	1	—	—	—	—	—	—
Nebr.	33	—	1	1	2	2	6	9	3	4	2	3	1
Kans.	31	1	1	4	—	3	6	2	6	2	—	4	2
S. Atlantic	1,680	4	13	27	35	136	357	254	216	115	118	193	212
Del.	26	—	—	—	1	2	10	5	5	—	—	2	1
Md.	311	—	1	4	9	22	93	55	50	21	26	29	1
D.C.	14	—	—	—	—	2	5	2	1	2	1	—	—
Va.	177	1	—	2	2	17	46	28	23	17	23	15	3
W. Va.	24	—	1	—	—	4	7	3	4	2	—	1	2

N.C.	171	1	—	2	4	20	33	35	28	18	15	15	—
S.C.	55	—	1	1	1	5	13	10	7	6	3	6	2
Ga.	193						NA						193
Fla.	709	2	10	18	18	64	150	116	98	49	50	124	10
E.S. Central	231	1	2	1	3	21	42	40	38	21	17	41	4
Ky.	46	1	—	1	1	7	12	10	4	6	2	1	1
Tenn.	76	—	1	—	1	6	8	9	15	7	11	18	—
Ala.	109	—	1	—	1	8	22	21	19	8	4	22	3
Miss.	—	—	—	—	—	—	—	—	—	—	—	—	—
W.S. Central	2,266	7	88	282	211	246	385	280	263	126	85	114	179
Ark.	89	—	2	5	3	14	10	14	11	6	6	7	11
La.	400	—	4	27	26	37	80	49	54	22	18	19	64
Okla.	169	—	4	15	10	20	34	28	15	12	8	11	12
Tex.	1,608	7	78	235	172	175	261	189	183	86	53	77	92
Mountain	1,057	11	52	91	70	110	209	159	156	67	38	38	56
Mont.	9	—	—	1	—	1	1	1	1	2	1	1	—
Idaho	3	—	—	—	—	—	—	1	—	—	—	—	2
Wyo.	29	—	1	—	3	4	8	2	6	2	3	—	—
Colo.	129	1	2	3	1	7	28	19	29	11	1	6	21
N. Mex.	61	2	7	7	4	9	6	10	6	4	3	2	1
Ariz.	530	7	29	60	38	59	101	73	76	29	19	21	18
Utah	151	1	10	15	20	20	24	21	16	11	6	4	3
Nev.	145	—	3	5	4	10	41	32	22	8	5	4	11
Pacific	2,787	—	87	202	156	323	637	471	400	180	123	134	74
Wash.	168	—	3	4	10	13	30	33	26	15	11	19	4
Oreg.	88	—	—	2	2	7	15	17	27	4	2	11	1
Calif.	2,488	—	84	194	141	300	580	415	339	158	108	100	69
Alaska	15	—	—	—	2	—	4	3	2	—	2	2	—
Hawaii	28	—	—	2	1	3	8	3	6	3	—	2	—
Guam	21	1	1	2	2	2	6	—	3	—	2	1	1
P.R.	163	—	4	20	23	32	27	20	14	8	5	5	5
V.I.	9	—	—	—	—	1	1	1	1	—	—	1	4
Pac. Trust Terr.	59						NA						59
C.N.M.I.	2						NA						2

*Does not include cases reported by state of Illinois
†Cases represent patients not tested for HBsAg
Source: *Atlanta Centers for Disease Control*

TABLE 3–4. Distribution of Viral Hepatitis Types A, B, and Non-A, Non-B, by Age, Sex, and Race, United States, 1981

AGE (YEARS)	PERCENTAGE OF CASES		
	Hepatitis A N = 4,151	Hepatitis B N = 9,130	Hepatitis B non-A, non-B N = 1,590
<5	4.4	0.6	1.5
5–9	8.0	0.7	2.6
10–14	6.7	0.7	3.2
15–19	9.3	11.1	7.4
20–29	33.7	47.9	34.8
30–39	17.1	18.6	17.1
40–49	7.2	8.1	9.4
50–59	6.0	5.8	7.0
≥60	7.7	6.3	17.0
Sex			
Male	57.2	62.7	53.2
Female	42.8	37.3	46.8
Race			
White	87.6	71.2	83.3
Black	6.0	20.5	11.5
Other	6.4	8.3	5.2

Source: *National Surveillance of Viral Hepatitis*, 1981

atitis B infection is only 10%; the probability of becoming a chronic carrier of the virus is less than 1%. In these regions, those at high risk are homosexuals, I.V. drug users, and blood-transfusion recipients. In the rest of the world, the lifetime risk of infection is between 20% and 40%. Chronic carrier risk is placed at between 2% and 5%.

Case control studies show that persistent HBV infection is significantly more common in PHC patients than in controls. Eighty percent of PHC arises in livers that either are cirrhotic or show signs of being actively inflamed, or both. The results of serologic testing in PHC patients and controls in several countries are summarized in Table 3–6.

To test if chronic hepatitis leads to PHC indirectly by causing cirrhosis, investigators in Japan studied patients with hepatitis B who had cirrhosis and cirrhotic patients who tested negative for HBsAg. The rate of PHC incidence for 4 years was 25% in those

TABLE 3–5.   Epidemiologic and Clinical Characteristics of Reported Cases of Viral Hepatitis by Serologic Type, 1981

EPIDEMIOLOGIC CHARACTERISTICS	Hepatitis A N = 4,151 No.	(%)	Hepatitis B N = 9,130 No.	(%)	Hepatitis non-A,non-B N = 1,591 No.	(%)
Child/employee in day-care center	247	(6)	57	(*)	41	(3)
Household contact of child/ employee in day-care center	381	(9)	161	(2)	71	(4)
Personal contact with hepatitis A	1,054	(25)	189	(2)	85	(5)
Employed as a food handler	274	(7)	476	(5)	71	(4)
Associated with food-borne or water-borne outbreak	164	(4)	87	(1)	19	(1)
International travel	207	(5)	126	(1)	35	(2)
Personal contact with hepatitis B	77	(2)	1,323	(14)	80	(5)
Employed in medical/dental field	103	(3)	683	(8)	113	(7)
Associated with dialysis/ transplant unit	12	(*)	202	(2)	29	(2)
Patient	7		92		12	
Employee	2		44		7	
Contact of patient/employee	2		49		7	
Blood transfusion	45	(1)	370	(4)	170	(11)
Hospitalized prior to illness	189	(5)	1,295	(14)	344	(22)
Surgery	81	(2)	617	(7)	180	(11)
Dental work	206	(5)	1,287	(14)	216	(14)
Drug abuse	79	(2)	1,133	(12)	131	(8)
Homosexual activity	93	(2)	512	(6)	32	(2)
Other percutaneous exposures	166	(4)	1,333	(15)	202	(13)
Clinical Characteristics						
Jaundice	3,161	(76)	6,262	(69)	1,025	(64)
Hospitalized for hepatitis	1,703	(41)	4,259	(47)	852	(54)
Death as a result of hepatitis	27	(*)	113	(1)	41	(3)

Source: *Atlanta Centers For Disease Control*

patients whose cirrhosis was related to the hepatitis B antigen compared to 6% in those whose cirrhosis was not related to hepatitis B.[a]

MORTALITY

The mortality from hepatitis infection worldwide is a major health problem because of the propensity of chronic infection to deteriorate to liver cirrhosis and PHC. In the United States, where the

[a]Obata H. Hepatitis B virus and liver cancer and cirrhosis of the liver. *Clinician* 24:63, 1977.

TABLE 3–6. Frequency of Hepatitis B Surface Antigen (HBsAG) and Antibody Against Hepatitis B Core (anti-HBc) in Blood of Patients with Primary Hepatic Carcinoma and in Controls in Selected Countries*

| COUNTRY | SERUMS OF PATIENTS WITH PRIMARY HEPATIC CARCINOMA | | SERUMS OF CONTROLS | |
	Number Tested	Percent Positive	Number Tested	Percent Positive
	Hepatitis B surface antigen			
Greece	189	55.0	106	4.7
Japan	260	37.3	4,387	2.6
Mozambique	29	62.1	35	14.3
Senegal	291	51.9	100	12.0
Singapore	156	35.3	1,516	4.1
South Africa	138	59.5	200	9.0
Spain	31	19.3	101	2.0
Taiwan	84	54.8	278	12.2
Uganda	47	47.0	50	6.0
United States	34	14.7	56	0
Vietnam	61	08.3	94	24.5
Zambia	19	63.1	40	7.5
	Antibody to hepatitis B core antigen			
Greece	80	70.0	160	31.9
Hong Kong	37	70.3	58	36.2
Senegal	291	87.3	100	26.0
South Africa	76	86.0	103	31.7
Spain	31	87.0	101	14.8
United States	33	48.5	56	0

*Table is based on studies using radiommunoassay or a test of equivalent sensitivity for HBsAG and in which controls were included
Source: *Public Health Reports*, Vol. 95, No. 5; 1980, p. 431

incidence of hepatitis is relatively low and where chronic infection is even less common, the annual number of deaths from hepatitis, including PHC deaths, is about 7,000. Death can also follow acute episodes of infection as well and accounts for annual mortality of nearly 1,000. The mortality rate during the 1980s is shown in Table 3–7.

The mortality rate from hepatitis by age is shown in Table 3–8.

PREVENTION

Because of the gravity of the disease and its high endemicity around the world, the development of the hepatitis B vaccine in 1981 was a major achievement in the battle against morbidity and death. Ini-

TABLE 3–7. Viral Hepatitis Mortality, United States 1980–84

DEATH RATE	1980	1981	1982	1983	1984
Number	790	760	840	840	810
Rate/100,000	0.03	0.03	0.04	0.04	0.04

Source: *Monthly Vital Statistics Report,* 32, 33; Nos. 9, 12, 13; September 1984, December 1984, March 1985

TABLE 3–8. Viral Hepatitis Mortality by Age, United States 1982

AGE (IN YEARS)	NUMBER	RATE/100,000
All ages	814	
Under 1	12	0.03
1–4	13	0.01
5–14	5	0.00
15–24	60	0.1
25–34	88	0.2
35–44	62	0.2
45–54	107	0.5
55–64	160	0.7
65–74	165	1.0
75–84	105	1.3

Source: *Monthly Vital Statistics Report,* Vol. 33, No. 9 Supplement, December 20, 1984

tial vaccine trials show the vaccine to be effective in preventing hepatitis B in 85% to 95% of those inoculated who develop antibodies to the virus. It became generally available in 1982. The CDC and the vaccine's manufacturer, Merck, Sharp and Dohme, have collected information on illnesses that developed in those receiving the vaccine.

In about 200,000 vaccinated subjects, 118 developed illness as of 1 March 1983; of these, 47.5% were ruled as unrelated to the vaccine for various reasons. Of the remaining 62 illnesses, 91.9% were reactions that fell into six primary classifications. They included neurologic problems, such as tremor and Bell's palsy, skin or mucous membrane lesions, such as hives or psoriasis, musculoskeletal ailments, including generalized aches, hepatitis-like symptoms, flu-like symptoms, and injection site reactions. Other symptoms included headache, vomiting, and self-limiting chest pain. Six patients had serious reactions for which they were hospitalized. These reactions included erythema multiforme, aseptic meningitis, grand mal seizure, and Guillain-Barré syndrome. The last-mentioned developed within 10 days of the patient's receiving the vaccine.

Since the vaccine is made from human blood plasma, there is some concern that it might carry the AIDS virus to vaccinees. As of this writing, however, no AIDS has been reported except in those patients already belonging to high-risk AIDS groups. Only homosexual male hospital workers, among the original vaccine recipients, have developed AIDS.

The vaccine was also tested for other well-known viruses often found in plasma. All indications show that the manufacturing process had inactivated all known viruses for which this check was done. Vaccine testing continues in high-risk hepatitis B groups, such as health-care workers, infants born to carrier mothers, staff members of institutions for the retarded, and Alaskan Eskimos, a group at high risk for the disease.

Practical distribution of the vaccine is being hampered at present, however, by the high cost of each three-dose regimen, which is $100. The vaccine, made from human plasma, is expensive particularly for use in areas where it is most needed and where annual per capita health expenditures are often less than $1. Even in the United States, some immunization programs have been possible only through funding from specific health grants.

Type A hepatitis is also endemic in underdeveloped countries where it is a common childhood disease. The virus was isolated in 1973, and detection tests were developed. Efforts to perfect a vaccine have taken longer, but the virus has been cultivated in cell culture. Now an attenuated hepatitis A virus (HAV) vaccine is being tested in human beings.

In western countries, those at risk for developing hepatitis A through contact with either an infected person or a contaminated food or water source are given immunoglobulin as soon as possible, and no later than 2 weeks after exposure. A 1979 study on the therapeutic effects of immunoglobulin was conducted in New Mexico where type A hepatitis incidence was high. The study showed that morbidity was reduced and health resources were saved by early intervention (Table 3–9).

CIRRHOSIS

Chronic hepatitis B can cause cirrhosis of the liver. Cirrhosis is a degenerative liver condition, causing fatty infiltration of liver tissue and changes in fibrous connective tissue. Initially, the liver becomes enlarged and smooth. Then as fibrous tissue and even extra bile ducts proliferate, the texture of the liver becomes granular. Blood vessels become thick and dysfunctional, causing greatly decreased hepatic blood circulation and gastrointestinal hemorrhage as liver portal hypertension develops. Eventually, the liver

TABLE 3–9.   Costs and Benefits of Hepatitis A Surveillance and Control, New Mexico, January–June 1979

COSTS	
Central Office:	
Personnel (physician-epidemiologist, nurse-epidemiologist, secretary)	$19,625
Supplies, telephone, mailings	900
Local Health Office:	
Personnel (public-health nurses, clerks)	13,000
Supplies (includes IG—immunoglobulin), telephone	500
Total	$34,025
BENEFITS	
HA cases averted among household contacts = 123*	
Total savings = 123 cases × $1,353 per case†	$166,419
Benefit-to-cost ratio = $166,419 to $34,025, or 4.89 to 1‡	

*706 household contacts given IG 14 days or less after onset of illness in index patient. Cases averted is difference between expected cases without IG (0.20 × 706 = 141) and expected cases with IG (0.025 × 706 = 18).
†Estimated direct and indirect costs of an HA case in 1979, based on data of Tolsma and Bryan *(11)* and updated to 1979 with 10% annual inflation factor.
‡Additional assumptions: *(a)* no beneficial effect to the 175 contacts given IG more than 14 days after onset in index patient, *(b)* no additional benefits from health department's work, such as more rapid patient diagnosis because of attention given HA, and *(c)* 87% protective efficacy of IG against symptomatic HA.
Source: *Public Health Reports,* Vol. 97, No. 6, 1982; p. 519

shrinks, its structure disintegrates, and scar tissue replaces fatty areas.

The disorder impairs liver function because normal liver cells die. In advanced stages of cirrhosis, the patient often dies of coma, jaundice, infection, high blood pressure, and hemorrhage. Coma results from chemical imbalances in the brain caused by a lack of liver function. Hepatic coma begins as general drowsiness and confusion and deteriorates to loss of consciousness.

In addition to chronic hepatitis B virus, cirrhosis can result from chronic alcohol consumption; inflammation of the bile ducts; congestive heart failure, causing liver congestion; protein malnutrition, especially in childhood; syphilis; animal parasite or viral infection; and exposure to toxic chemicals, such as carbon tetrachloride. Cirrhosis may also develop from excessive iron or copper deposits in the liver.

The most common cause of liver cirrhosis in North America is excessive alcohol consumption. This form is sometimes called Laennec's cirrhosis. A decade ago, the prevailing explanation for the connection between excessive alcohol consumption and cirrhosis was that nutritional deficits common among alcoholics caused the liver to degenerate. Efforts, albeit unsuccessful, have been made by the medical community to have vitamins added to alcoholic beverages, since the latter have no substantive nutritional or vitamin content but represent rather, empty calories. Investigators are beginning to hypothesize that alcohol itself has a direct, harmful effect on the liver which can be stopped only by abstinence. Even social drinking can be harmful.[b]

Currently, cirrhosis and chronic hepatic diseases rank as the ninth leading cause of death in the United States. Data collected on this cause of death do not show much disruption between the various revisions of the International Classification of Disease. The comparability ratio between the Sixth and Seventh Revisions is 0.99, whereas the ratio between the Seventh and Eighth is 1.0055. Thus, mortality changes reflect actual changes that have occurred as of the 1970s. The death rate due to cirrhosis peaked in 1973 at 15.9 deaths per 100,000. By 1977, the rate had dropped to 14.3 and by 1984 the rate was 11.4.

The rise in mortality that took place between 1960 and 1973 for people of both sexes and major racial groups was not due to age distribution changes in the populations. These dramatic increases amounted to 31% for white males—up from 15.6 to 20.5 per 100,000, and 36% for white women, a rise from 7.4 to 10.1. But, the truly amazing jump in mortality occurred among blacks during this time. The rate for nonwhite males rose 111%, from 12.6 to 26.7 per 100,000 and 92% for nonwhite women, rising from 7.9 to 15.2 deaths per 100,000.

The trend in death rate for people by age, sex, and race and the age-adjusted death rate for all of them between 1960 and 1984 are shown in Table 3–10. The white population, which has lower cirrhosis death rates in general than the black population, showed more modest mortality increases than blacks until 1973 and a greater mortality decline after 1973.

Cirrhosis deaths related to alcohol consumption as reported during the Eighth Revision, 1968–1977, accounted for 121,256 deaths. This was 38.4% of all deaths from cirrhosis for the entire 10-year period. The percentage of alcohol-related cirrhosis increased during these 10 years as well, rising from 34.4% in 1968 to 42.2% in 1977. This percentage breakdown for cirrhosis from different causes, including alcohol consumption in 1968 and 1977, is shown in Table 3–11.

The mortality rate due to chronic liver disease and cirrhosis in several countries, as of latest reported year, is shown in Table 3–12.

Epidemiologists are not positing definitive explanations for the decline that seems to be taking place in mortality since 1973, but

---

[b]Sherlock S. *Alcohol and the Liver in Diseases of the Liver and Biliary System*, 5th ed. Oxford: Blackwell, pp. 445–460, 1975.

several factors may be causative. Alcohol consumption increased in the United States in the 1970s, and early 1980s. Still, data suggest that the increased consumption is due to more drinking among a subset of drinkers; other drinkers are moving toward either abstinence or lowered consumption. Thus, intensity is replacing breadth in alcohol consumption. This trend may result in fewer deaths from cirrhosis.

Development of the hepatitis B vaccine in 1981 and the determination in 1975 that non-A, non-B hepatitis could be transmitted by blood transfusion, together with the development of tests to identify hepatitis B in blood products, may also be reducing cirrhosis mortality in the last 12 years.

Another major life-saving advance, developed in the past 20 years, is the liver transplant. It was first performed in 1963. The survival rates reported in two recent series range from 28% to 70%. Several post-transplant patients are leading normal lives, especially since the advent of cyclosporin A, a lungal metabolite that has increased survival by 1 year in a large number of patients. The University of Tennesee and the University of Minnesota are also developing programs for liver transplant.

As with other transplant programs, lack of suitable organs still poses one of the greatest difficulties for patients. Generally, this lack prohibits HLA-type matching between donor and patient. It does not seem to be an obstacle to success, however, since the rejection phenomenon is not as pronounced in liver transplant procedures as it is in others. Still, an estimated 28% of children who need a new liver do not qualify for a transplant because of hepatic structural anomalies, such as an absent infrahepatic vena cava. Some side effects in children who receive liver transplants are cystic-duct stenosis or stone formation and biliary-tract complications.

The demographic pattern of liver disease, including cirrhosis, shows a higher incidence in males at all ages than in females, higher in middle-aged than in young patients, and higher in those with low incomes (Table 3–13, pp. 76–77).

LIVER DISEASE DISABILITY

The years of potential life lost before age 65 years by persons dying in 1981 of chronic liver disease and cirrhosis amounted to 267,350. The estimated number of physician contacts needed to treat liver diseases in 1982 was 107,000.

TABLE 3–10. Death Rates for Cirrhosis of Liver by Age, Race, and Sex and Corresponding Age-adjusted Rates. United States, 1960–77, Overall 1982–84 (For 1968–77 rates are based on deaths assigned to category number 571 of the *Eighth Revision International Classification of Diseases, Adapted for Use in the United States, 1965* [ICDA]; 1960–67 rates are based on deaths assigned to category number 581 of the Seventh Revision adopted in 1955)

RACE, SEX, AND YEAR	All Ages	25–34 Years	35–44 Years	45–54 Years	55–64 Years	65–74 Years	75–84 Years	85 Years and Over	Age-Adjusted Rate
Both sexes				Rate per 100,000 population					
1984	11.4								
1983	11.9								
1982	11.9								
1977*	14.3	3.8	15.3	33.8	45.4	42.6	30.2	16.9	13.1
1976*	14.7	3.7	16.9	35.0	47.6	42.6	29.3	18.0	13.6
1975*	14.8	3.8	16.7	36.0	49.0	42.8	29.0	16.9	13.8
1974*	15.8	4.2	18.6	38.7	50.9	45.9	29.5	18.6	14.8
1973*	15.9	4.2	19.4	39.1	52.5	44.6	28.8	19.9	15.0
1972* †	15.6	4.3	20.3	38.9	50.3	43.1	29.5	20.3	14.9
1971*	15.4	4.2	19.3	38.5	49.8	42.2	30.1	21.6	14.7
1970*	15.5	4.4	19.6	38.3	49.3	42.2	30.9	20.3	14.7
1969	14.8	4.3	19.0	36.7	47.2	39.8	29.5	21.5	14.1
1968	14.6	4.2	18.1	36.8	46.1	40.3	29.6	22.7	13.9
1967	14.1	4.0	17.1	35.1	45.2	39.7	28.1	22.6	13.4
1966	13.6	3.8	16.6	34.1	42.9	38.4	30.5	24.2	13.0
1965	12.8	3.5	15.0	32.2	39.8	36.7	30.5	21.5	12.1
1964	12.1	3.3	13.9	29.8	38.0	35.6	29.9	25.3	11.4
1963	11.9	3.3	12.7	30.1	36.3	36.6	29.9	26.1	11.2
1962	11.7	3.2	13.0	29.0	35.4	36.5	29.7	26.3	11.0
1961	11.3	3.1	12.3	27.5	34.2	35.3	30.2	25.9	10.6
1960	11.3	2.9	11.8	27.6	32.7	37.4	32.1	28.8	10.5
White, male									
1982	15.8								
1977*	18.3	3.4	16.1	41.2	62.1	64.0	48.2	28.6	16.7
1976*	18.9	3.2	17.8	43.3	65.4	65.6	46.5	31.0	17.5
1975*	19.3	3.2	18.3	44.7	66.8	67.4	47.2	28.6	17.9

Year									
1974*	20.4	3.5	19.2	47.7	69.7	73.4	48.1	30.2	19.0
1973*	20.5	3.6	20.0	47.9	73.4	70.7	45.7	32.9	19.3
1972*,†	20.2	3.3	21.3	48.0	71.5	66.8	46.2	36.1	19.1
1971*	20.1	3.5	20.0	47.9	71.3	66.0	47.3	35.7	18.9
1970*	20.1	3.4	19.7	47.3	70.6	67.8	48.1	33.1	18.8
1969	19.2	3.3	19.2	45.3	68.2	62.1	45.2	36.4	18.0
1968	18.9	3.0	18.8	45.1	66.2	62.5	45.9	32.6	17.7
1967	18.3	3.0	18.1	43.4	64.6	61.7	42.4	33.1	17.2
1966	17.8	2.5	17.3	42.3	62.9	60.0	46.4	38.6	16.7
1965	16.6	2.5	15.2	39.8	57.7	57.4	48.4	32.5	15.6
1964	16.0	2.5	14.3	38.0	54.9	57.2	45.8	36.1	15.0
1963‡	15.7	2.5	13.2	38.0	52.3	58.2	44.4	37.8	14.7
1962‡	15.7	2.5	13.6	38.1	51.7	56.6	44.8	39.6	14.6
1961	15.4	2.5	13.3	35.9	50.3	56.6	47.0	34.8	14.2
1960	15.6	2.3	13.4	36.5	49.2	59.7	46.8	41.7	14.4
White, female									
1982	8.2								
1977*	9.1	1.3	7.5	19.4	27.0	27.7	20.1	13.0	7.5
1976*	9.3	1.3	8.1	20.4	28.7	25.8	20.5	13.7	7.7
1975*	9.4	1.3	7.9	21.6	30.2	24.8	19.2	11.9	7.9
1974*	10.0	1.7	9.8	22.9	31.4	26.4	19.2	14.0	8.6
1973‡	10.1	1.6	10.1	24.0	31.8	25.8	19.2	14.3	8.7
1972*,†	9.9	1.6	10.3	23.6	30.2	25.2	20.5	13.1	8.6
1971*	10.0	1.7	10.6	24.1	30.0	25.3	20.5	15.3	8.7
1970*	10.0	1.6	10.8	24.7	29.6	24.1	21.2	15.4	8.7
1969	9.5	1.8	10.6	23.7	27.5	23.3	20.6	14.2	8.4
1968	9.6	1.8	10.4	23.8	27.6	24.5	20.2	18.8	8.5
1967	9.4	1.8	10.0	23.9	27.6	23.7	19.7	18.2	8.3
1966	8.9	1.8	9.9	22.7	24.4	22.8	20.8	17.0	7.9
1965	8.5	1.8	9.3	22.2	23.2	22.2	19.5	16.1	7.6
1964	8.2	1.7	9.3	20.4	23.2	20.4	19.8	21.1	7.3
1963‡	8.0	1.6	8.8	21.1	21.1	20.4	20.6	21.1	7.2
1962‡	7.6	1.7	9.0	18.9	19.7	20.3	19.6	19.7	6.8
1961	7.5	1.6	8.6	18.8	20.1	19.4	19.6	22.1	6.7
1960	7.4	1.8	8.2	18.1	18.0	20.8	22.7	22.2	6.6

TABLE 3–10 (Continued).

All other, male

RACE, SEX, AND YEAR	All Ages	25-34 Years	35-44 Years	45-54 Years	55-64 Years	65-74 Years	75-84 Years	85 Years and Over	Age-Adjusted Rate
				Rate per 100,000 population					
1982	16.6								
1977*	24.9	18.3	55.2	87.5	88.9	50.3	35.0	11.1	31.4
1976*	25.4	18.6	61.2	86.3	90.7	54.0	23.5	8.8	32.3
1975*	25.3	20.1	57.4	86.1	89.1	56.3	33.0	17.2	32.1
1974*	26.7	20.9	65.1	93.6	88.3	54.7	31.5	12.3	34.0
1973*	26.6	20.8	68.4	88.8	86.4	54.0	31.0	35.8	33.9
1972*,†	27.5	21.0	70.2	96.9	81.8	62.8	30.6	27.5	36.1
1971*	24.4	20.2	63.1	82.8	73.0	51.6	29.2	20.4	31.1
1970*	24.6	22.7	65.6	82.6	71.3	47.5	24.9	9.0	31.3
1969	24.2	20.0	65.3	75.4	73.8	52.1	23.9	25.0	30.6
1968	23.0	21.0	54.4	81.1	67.9	46.9	25.8	14.6	29.0
1967	21.2	17.8	55.1	64.7	60.8	49.8	29.3	30.8	26.4
1966	20.8	19.8	50.8	65.5	60.1	46.9	26.8	30.6	26.0
1965	18.5	15.0	45.7	59.5	57.1	36.2	27.3	23.5	22.9
1964	15.7	12.0	37.5	49.7	49.2	32.9	30.2	9.4	19.3
1963‡	13.9	11.1	31.8	39.4	47.0	34.0	24.8	17.2	16.9
1962‡	13.9	10.2	31.5	38.6	45.3	34.8	25.5	31.0	16.7
1961	13.3	12.0	27.3	38.5	41.1	33.9	21.4	10.0	16.9
1960	12.6	9.3	23.8	39.1	41.5	30.9	23.3	22.3	14.9

All other, female

Year									
1982	9.1								
1977*	12.9	9.6	27.1	42.1	38.4	22.3	18.3	6.8	15.0
1976*	13.1	8.9	30.7	41.6	38.1	24.9	14.5	5.0	15.4
1975*	13.2	9.8	30.7	40.8	39.8	24.4	11.5	11.8	15.5
1974*	14.7	11.6	34.3	48.7	42.2	22.2	14.0	8.2	17.4
1973*	15.2	11.7	36.8	51.0	41.3	25.1	14.4	1.1	18.0
1972*,†	14.4	14.6	39.1	43.8	33.5	22.9	9.2	7.3	17.2
1971*	14.2	12.3	37.5	46.2	34.6	20.0	12.2	11.8	16.9
1970*	14.6	14.2	40.5	43.4	34.6	20.7	15.4	3.8	17.4
1969	14.3	14.2	38.1	45.8	32.3	19.6	13.8	12.3	17.1
1968	13.9	13.5	37.8	44.3	29.7	18.2	10.0	11.5	16.6
1967	12.2	14.0	30.8	37.2	30.8	16.4	6.9		14.6
1966	12.3	12.1	32.5	38.4	30.2	15.0	11.8	9.4	14.7
1965	11.1	11.8	30.7	31.0	26.4	14.0	10.3	10.2	13.2
1964	9.5	11.5	26.2	25.5	19.5	12.0	10.7	8.9	11.2
1963‡	9.3	12.0	21.0	27.3	21.5	14.0	8.9	14.3	10.9
1962‡	9.3	11.3	21.3	26.9	20.9	15.8	11.4	7.5	10.9
1961	8.4	9.8	21.3	23.4	18.6	12.2	8.9	15.0	9.8
1960	7.9	9.0	18.5	23.1	17.1	11.5	13.1	14.9	9.1

*Excludes deaths of nonresidents of the United States
†Based on a 50% sample of deaths
‡Figures by race exclude data for residents of New Jersey because this state did not require reporting of the item for these years
Source: *Vital and Health Statistics*, Series 17, Vol. 20

TABLE 3–11. Number and Percentage Distribution of Deaths from Cirrhosis of Liver by Subcategories Alcoholic, Other Specified, and Unspecified, According to Race and Sex: United States, 1968 and 1977 (numbers after causes of death are category numbers of the *Eighth Revision International Classification of Diseases, Adapted for Use in the United States, 1965 (ICDA)*)

YEAR, RACE, AND SEX	Cirrhosis of Liver (571)	Alcoholic (571.0)	Other Specified (†571.8)*	Unspecified (†571.9)*	Cirrhosis of Liver (571)	Alcoholic (571.0)	Other Specified (571.8)*	Unspecified (571.9)*
	Number of deaths				Percent distribution			
1977								
Total	30,848	13,029	3,908	13,911	100.0	42.2	12.7	45.1
White, male	16,727	7,241	1,658	7,828	100.0	43.3	9.9	46.8
White, female	8,721	3,102	1,343	4,276	100.0	35.6	15.4	49.0
All other, male	3,440	1,791	554	1,095	100.0	52.1	16.1	31.8
All other, female	1,960	895	353	712	100.0	45.7	18.0	36.3
1968								
Total	29,183	10,036	5,694	13,453	100.0	34.4	19.5	46.1
White, male	16,142	5,738	2,739	7,665	100.0	35.5	17.0	47.5
White, female	8,607	2,511	1,918	4,178	100.0	29.2	22.3	48.5
All other, male	2,679	1,135	591	953	100.0	42.4	22.1	35.6
All other, female	1,755	552	446	657	100.0	37.2	25.4	37.4

*The Eighth Revision adapted for use in the United States has the three subcategories shown in the report, whereas the Revision adopted by the World Health Organization has only two subcategories: Alcoholic (ICD No. 571.0) and Other (ICD No. 571.9). The inclusion terms under the three subcategories in use in the United States are as follows:

571.0 Alcoholic   *571.8 Other specified   *571.9 Unspecified

Alcoholic:
cirrhosis
hepatitis
Laennec's cirrhosis
Any condition in 571.8 or 571.9
with mention of alcohol or
alcoholism

Cirrhosis (hepatic)
(liver):
biliary
cardiac
congenital
due to passive
congestion
portal
postnecrotic
Fatty degeneration
of liver
} Without mention of alcohol or alcoholism

Banti's disease
Chronic hepatitis
Cirrhosis (hepatic)
(liver):
NOS
hepatolienal
splenomegalic
Hepatolienal fibrosis
} Without mention or alcohol or alcoholism

The ICDA gives greater detail and specificity than is provided by the Eighth Revision of the ICD. Complete correspondence between these two classifications has been maintained at the three digit level, but new fourth-digit subdivisions have been renumbered to accommodate the additional subcategories in logical sequence. Those subdivisions of the ICDA which do not correspond exactly with the ICD are identified by an asterisk (*). This explains the asterisks in this table before 571.8 and 571.9. The † is also used, as is described in tables 8, A, B, C, K, L, and M, to identify titles that were introduced by the National Center for Health Statistics after the publication of ICDA.
Source: *Vital and Health Statistics*, Series 20, Vol. 17

TABLE 3–12. Mortality Rate per 100,000 due to Chronic Liver Disease and Cirrhosis of the Liver for Several Countries by Latest Reported Year

COUNTRY	RATE	YEAR
Costa Rica	6.0	1981
Guatemala	6.0	1980
Chile	29.6	1980
Israel	7.8	1980
Japan	14.1	1980
Kuwait	3.8	1979
Austria	29.3	1981
Bulgaria	11.4	1981
France	28.2	1980
Greece	11.3	1981
Hungary	27.7	1980
Poland	12.3	1980
United Kingdom		
England, Wales	4.5	1981
Australia	8.4	1981
United States	11.4	1982

Source: *U.N. Demographic Yearbook, 1982*

The discharged patients and the average hospital stay for patients with these diseases in different parts of the country in 1980 is shown in Table 3–14.

The patients hospitalized and the hospitalization rate of patients with chronic liver disease and cirrhosis in 1980 according to age and sex is shown in Table 3–15.

TABLE 3–14. Geographic Distribution of Discharged Patients, Rate and Average Length of Stay in Short-term Hospitals United States 1980 (Chronic Liver Disease and Cirrhosis ICDA. 571)

CHRONIC LIVER DISEASE AND CIRRHOSIS	ALL	NORTHEAST	NORTH CENTRAL	SOUTH	WEST
Patients (in 1,000s)	115	33	28	33	21
Rate/10,000 population	6.7	6.6	7.4	7.0	5.2
Average length of stay	8.9	9.1	9.2	8.7	8.8

Source: *National Hospital Discharge Survey, 1980*

TABLE 3–15. Patients Hospitalized, United States, 1980 for Chronic Liver Disease and Cirrhosis by Age and Sex

PATIENTS HOSPITALIZED	ALL AGES	UNDER 15	15–44	45–64	65+
Rate/100,000	14.8	7.8	36.0	36.8	36.8
Number in 1,000s		Male 197		Female 134	
Rate		18.3		11.6	

Source: *National Hospital Discharge Survey, 1980*

TABLE 3–13. Number and Rate per 1,000 Population of Liver Conditions Reported in Health Interviews, by Age and Selected Characteristics: United States, 1975 (data are based on household interviews of the civilian noninstitutionalized population)

CHARACTERISTICS	Number of conditions in thousands					Rate per 1,000 population				
	ALL AGES	UNDER 45 YEARS		45–64 YEARS	65 YEARS AND OVER	ALL AGES	UNDER 45 YEARS		45–64 YEARS	65 YEARS AND OVER
		Total	17–44 Years				Total	17–44 Years		
Total	411	142	122	189	79	2.0	1.0	1.5	4.4	3.7
Sex										
Male	231	74	65	117	40	2.3	1.0	1.6	5.7	4.6
Female	179	68	56	72	40	1.7	0.9	1.3	3.2	3.2
Race										
White	366	120	99	170	76	2.0	1.0	1.4	4.4	3.9
All other	45	22*	22*	19*	3*	1.7	1.1*	2.0*	4.3*	1.5*
Black	45	22*	22*	19*	3*	1.8	1.2*	2.3*	4.7*	1.6*
Usual activity status										
School age (6–16 years)	17*	17*	—	—	—	0.4*	0.4*	—	—	—
Usually working (17 years and over)	141	64	64	72	5*	1.8	1.3	1.3	2.7	2.0*
Usually keeping house (female, 17 years and over)	100	27*	27*	40	32*	2.5	1.5*	1.5*	3.3	3.1*
Retired (45 years and over)	80	—	—	48	32*	8.2	—	—	20.4	4.3*
Other activity (17 years and over)	69	31*	31*	29*	9*	4.0	2.1*	2.1*	19.6*	8.6*
Marital status										
Married	215	57	57	122	36	2.2	1.1	1.1	3.5	3.1
Formerly married	129	31*	31*	54	43	6.1	5.0*	5.0*	8.4	5.1
Widowed	63	5*	5*	25*	33*	5.5	10.3*	10.3*	7.4*	4.3*
Separated	19*	11*	11*	7*	2*	5.8*	5.2*	5.2*	7.6*	8.2*
Divorced	46	16*	16*	22*	8*	7.3	4.4*	4.4*	10.4*	14.4*
Never Married	47	33*	33*	14*	—	1.7	1.3*	1.3*	6.1*	—

Employment status										
In the labor force (17 years and over)										
Employed	176	81	81	82	12*	1.9	1.4	1.4	2.9	4.0*
Unemployed	144	65	65	68	11*	1.7	1.2	1.2	2.5	3.9*
	32*	17*	17*	14*	2*	4.0*	2.8*	2.8*	8.6*	9.5*
Not in the labor force (17 years and over)	215	40	40	107	67	3.8	1.7	1.7	7.2	3.7
Living arrangements										
Living alone	84	20*	20*	44	21*	5.5	3.7*	3.8*	10.5	3.6*
Living with nonrelatives	12*	2*	2*	7*	3*	3.3	0.7*	0.7*	14.3*	9.5*
Living with spouse	213	57	57	120	36	2.2	1.1	1.1	3.5	3.2
Living with other relatives	101	63	43	19*	19*	1.1	0.7	1.8	4.4*	5.1*
Family income										
Less than $5,000	134	42	39	66	25*	4.2	2.3	3.8	12.4	3.0*
$5,000–$9,999	111	32*	28*	47	33*	2.5	1.0*	1.6*	5.4	5.6*
$10,000–$14,999	69	28*	24*	32*	7*	1.5	0.8*	1.2*	3.7*	3.3*
$15,000 or more	70	27*	18*	34*	9*	1.0	0.5*	0.6*	2.2*	3.7*
Education of head of family										
Less than 12 years	227	71	62	104	53	3.0	1.6	2.7	5.5	4.0
12 years	100	41	33*	41	18*	1.5	0.8	1.1*	3.2	4.5*
13–15 years	35	16*	14*	14*	5*	1.2	0.7*	1.0*	3.0*	3.0*
16 years or more	46	12*	10*	31*	4*	1.4	0.5*	0.7*	5.3*	2.2*
Place of residence										
SMSA	279	97	88	136	47	1.9	1.0	1.5	4.6	3.5
Central city	148	47	42	75	26*	2.4	1.1	1.7	5.8	3.9*
Outside central city	131	49	46	61	21*	1.6	0.8	1.4	3.6	3.1*
Outside SMSA	131	45	34*	53	33*	2.0	1.0	1.4*	4.0	4.2*
Nonfarm	118	35	27*	53	29*	2.0	0.9	1.2*	4.0	4.2*
Farm	14*	10*	7*	—	3*	2.1*	2.5*	3.2*	—	3.5*
Region										
Northeast	84	17*	15*	49	17*	1.7	0.5*	0.8*	4.5	3.2*
North Central	104	38	33*	52	15*	1.9	1.0	1.5*	4.7	2.6*
South	135	50	43	51	34*	2.0	1.1	1.6	3.8	5.1*
West	88	38	31*	37	13*	2.4	1.4	2.0*	4.9	3.9*

*May not be reliable
Source: *Vital and Health Statistics*, Series 10, No. 115

4 Diabetes

DIABETES

Diabetes is the most common metabolic disease in the United States. According to the American Diabetes Association, there were 12 million diabetics in 1985.

Diabetes amounts to a state of chronic hyperglycemia and disturbances of carbohydrate and lipid metabolism. It often leads to several secondary pathologic conditions, including blindness and cardiovascular disease.

Several types of diabetes are known. Some researchers believe that each may be a distinct disease. Although the underlying cause of diabetes is unknown, one immediate cause is failure of the pancreatic islands of Langerhans to manufacture insulin in response to elevated serum glucose levels. But it is also suspected that occasionally diabetes results from a loss of receptors needed for insulin utilization. The liver uses insulin to absorb glucose from the bloodstream and stores it as glycogen. Diabetic acidosis is a dangerous condition threatening uncontrolled diabetics. It develops when the liver is unable to absorb glucose and starts to manufacture it by breaking down fat. Fatty acids build up in the bloodstream and cause the acidosis that can lead to diabetic coma.

The earliest occurring type of diabetes with onset typically in children 10- to 14-years old is *juvenile-onset diabetes*. Onset is sudden, and those with this form are usually insulin dependent. They need daily insulin supplements to control their serum glucose level. They are generally subject to more illness than those with the second major type, type II diabetes—*maturity-onset diabetes.* The latter develops most typically after age 40 years. Generally its onset is gradual and insidious. But its effects can often be controlled through diet without the need for exogenous insulin.

Another diabetes syndrome that occurs in pregnant women is *gestational diabetes.* Although it usually disappears after delivery, a high percentage of gestational diabetics become maturity onset diabetics within 16 years of their first pregnancy.

Symptoms of types I and II include increased thirst, excessive urination, hunger, itching, weight loss, and—occasionally—dehydration and diabetic coma. The chief management problem is maintaining a balanced insulin and serum glucose level similar to physiologic levels. Too much insulin and the patient develops shock; too little and he develops diabetic coma (diabetic acidosis).

INCIDENCE AND PREVALENCE

The prevalence figures of diabetes are not altogether reliable because many diabetics do not know they have the disease in the early stages of development. Some diabetics are detected when their serum glucose levels become so high that sugar spills into their urine (glycosuria). But a person may be diabetic long before glycosuria develops. The most sensitive test for detecting diabetes is the glucose tolerance test.

The criterion for deciding that a person is diabetic is a 1-hour serum glucose level of 200 mg/dl or more after imbibing a 50-g oral glucose load. This standard is not universally accepted, however. Disagreement exists on how the results of the standard glucose tolerance test should be interpreted. In 1960, this standard was applied to the results of a probability sampling of the U.S. population. In addition to the 1.8% who knew they were diabetic through earlier diagnosis, an additional 3.9% of the sample population had glucose levels after 1 hour indicative of probable diabetes. The results extrapolated to the noninstitutionalized population equaled 2 million persons previously diagnosed and 4.25 million previously undetected. The total was well over 6 million diabetics nationwide as of 1960.

The prevalence of diabetes per 1,000 civilian noninstitutionalized population by age, race, sex, and other selected demographic characteristics obtained from the National Health Interview Survey for 1979–1981 is presented in Table 4–1. As can be seen, the

TABLE 4–1. Average Annual Number of Persons with Known Diabetes per 1,000 Population by Age and Selected Socio-demographic Characteristics: United States, 1979–81 (data are based on annual one-third subsamples of National Health Interview Survey household interviews of the civilian noninstitutionalized population)

| | | | AGE | | | | | |
| | | | | 17 Years and Over | | | 65 Years and Over | |
CHARACTERISTIC	All Ages	Under 17 Years	All Persons 17 Years and Over	17–44 Years	45–64 Years	All Persons 65 Years and Over	65–74 Years	75 Years and Over
			Number of persons with known diabetes per 1,000 population					
Total**	24.7	0.9	33.3	9.1	55.0	88.4	87.7	89.4
Sex								
Male	22.2	0.7*	30.7	7.7	55.0	85.1	87.9	79.3
Female	27.0	1.1*	35.7	10.4	55.1	90.7	87.7	95.3
Race								
White	23.8	1.0	31.6	8.5	49.9	84.3	83.4	86.0
All other	30.5	0.6*	45.9	12.8	97.4	127.7	128.4	126.5
Black	32.2	0.7*	48.8	14.5	99.9	129.8	129.3	130.9
Hispanic origin								
Hispanic	22.2	1.0*	33.1	9.4	88.7	84.9	84.5	85.6
Non-Hispanic	25.0	0.8	33.4	9.0	53.3	88.4	87.9	89.3
Education of individual								
Less than 12 years	...	...	57.0	11.7	77.7	104.0	104.7	102.9
12 years	...	...	25.0	8.5	48.9	65.6	69.6	56.0
More than 12 years	...	...	18.8	7.8	33.6	68.9	64.6	78.6

Marital status								
Married	⋯	⋯	34.2	10.4	50.5	90.9	91.4	89.5
Formerly married	⋯	⋯	60.9	14.0	77.7	89.4	87.6	91.1
Never married	⋯	⋯	10.3	5.2	52.9	56.8	47.3	72.9
Education of head of family								
Less than 12 years	41.0	0.5*	54.2	12.8	73.9	99.2	100.7	96.8
12 years	18.9	1.3*	25.9	7.7	50.9	72.9	71.5	75.9
More than 12 years	14.2	0.9*	19.0	7.5	33.0	72.6	68.1	81.5
Family income†								
Less than $7,000	45.0	0.8*	59.7	12.3	102.9	108.1	98.9	119.7
$7,000–$9,999	34.7	0.0*	45.9	11.0	90.0	72.1	80.7	54.7
$10,000–$14,999	27.2	2.9*	35.8	4.9	71.9	90.3	93.1	83.7
$15,000–$24,999	18.5	0.8*	25.9	9.7	44.4	96.7	89.1	115.2
$25,000 or more	16.4	1.8*	21.4	8.7	38.5	73.1	62.5	97.2
Location of residence								
SMSA‡	24.1	0.9	32.2	8.9	55.2	86.2	85.4	87.6
Central city	27.7	0.8*	36.8	10.0	65.9	86.9	88.2	84.9
Outside central city	21.6	1.0*	29.0	8.1	48.1	85.6	83.1	90.1
Outside SMSA‡	26.1	0.9*	35.8	9.5	54.6	92.2	92.0	92.7
Nonfarm	26.2	0.6*	36.2	10.0	56.4	92.5	90.2	96.5
Farm	24.9	5.2*	31.7	3.9*	39.8	89.7	109.5	52.5
Geographic region								
Northeast	24.9	0.8*	33.0	8.5	51.4	85.6	86.0	84.9
North Central	24.3	0.9*	33.0	9.6	55.1	86.8	78.8	100.1
South	27.5	1.2*	37.4	9.4	64.7	95.6	100.9	86.1
West	20.2	0.5*	27.2	8.4	42.2	80.7	77.9	85.6

*May be unreliable
**Includes unknown Hispanic origin, education of individual, marital status, education of head of family, and family income
†Data are for 1981 only, because information on annual family income is only available for broad income categories and is technically difficult to adjust for inflation over the 3-year time period
‡SMSA = standard metropolitan statistical area
Source: *National Center for Health Statistics: Computed by the Division of Epidemiology and Health Promotion from 1979–81 National Health Interview Survey data provided by the Division of Health Interview Statistics*

rates for non-whites are much higher than those for whites age 65 years or older. And black women, in particular, have a higher rate than men, the prevalence increasing with age. Until advanced age, diabetes rates are inversely proportional to a person's education level.

Before the 1979–81 survey, the prevalence of diabetes was measured in 1964–1965 and in 1972–1973. The change between the two earlier studies is shown in Tables 4–2 and 4–3. The overall prevalence rate increased from 14.5 per 1,000 to 20.4 per 1,000 persons between the earlier surveys, an increase of 41%. The rate increased 50% for females, jumping from 16.1 per 1,000 to 24.1 per

TABLE 4–2.   Changes in Prevalence of Reported Diabetes Among Males and Females by Age Between 1965–66 and 1973, Health Interview Survey, United States

	RATES/1,000 PERSONS		
SEX AND AGE	1965–66	1973	CHANGE (%)
All Persons	14.5	20.4	+41
Males:			
All ages	12.9	16.3	+26
<45	3.7	4.3	+16
45–64	29.6	40.6	+37
65+	51.4	60.3	+17
Females:			
All ages	16.1	24.1	+50
<45	3.8	6.8	+79
45–64	31.0	44.4	+43
65+	70.5	91.3	+29

Source: *Health Interview Survey 1965–66 and 1973*, National Center for Health Statistics

TABLE 4–3.   Changes in Prevalence of Reported Diabetes Among Whites and Non-Whites by Age Between 1964–65 and 1973, Health Interview Survey United States

	RATES/1,000 PERSONS		
RACE AND AGE	1964–65	1973	CHANGE (%)
White			
All ages	12.1	19.9	+64
<45	3.0	5.3	+77
45+	32.8	51.4	+57
Non-white			
All ages	13.3	23.9	+80
<45	2.8	7.0	+150
45+	50.2	80.3	+60

Source: *Health Interview Survey 1964–65 and 1973*, National Center for Health Statistics

1,000 and by 26% for males from 12.9 per 1,000 to 16.3 per 1,000. Increases were greatest among middle-aged men and women younger than age 45 years. The changes between 1973 and 1978 were equally notable, increasing from 20.4 per 1,000 in 1973 (Table 4–2) to 24.7 per 1,000 for the total population (Table 4–1).

The changes in diabetes prevalence between 1964–1965 and 1973 according to age and race are presented in Table 4–3. The increased prevalence is highest for non-whites younger than under age 45 years.

The annual reported incidence of diabetes rose from 325,000 in 1965 to 612,000 in 1973 and 691,000 in 1978. Some of the changes in both reported prevalence and incidence are no doubt related to increased awareness by the public and the medical community about undetected diabetes. Technologic advances during this time, such as automated blood chemistries, have also extended the availability of diagnostic testing.

RISK FACTORS

Heredity

Evidence from several studies indicates that diabetes is partly related to heredity and genetic endowment. This association has been noted in studies of twins and relatives of diabetics. These subjects have a higher prevalence of diabetes than the relatives of nondiabetics. But the picture is more complex than what these associations indicate. The mode of inheritance has not been identified, and the role it plays in the development of juvenile-onset diabetes and maturity-onset diabetes is thought to be different.

Juvenile type I diabetes seems to be related to certain HLA markers (human leukocyte antigens). But this does not seem to be true for maturity-onset diabetes, type II diabetes. But the rate of type II diabetes is six times higher in the siblings of type II diabetics than in the siblings of nondiabetic controls. Moreover, the children of type II diabetics are twice as likely to develop diabetes than are the children of age-matched nondiabetics. Gravidas who develop gestational diabetes also have a family history with greater prevalence of overt diabetes.

Obesity

Studies indicate that obesity is an important risk factor in the development of type II diabetes. When obese siblings of diabetic patients were compared with nonobese siblings of diabetic patients, the disease's prevalence among the obese siblings was

three times higher than among the others.[a] An interesting observation has also been made that 75% of obese hyperglycemic
patients show a return to normal glucose tolerance when they lose
weight.[b] Obese women of all ages also show a twofold increased
risk for gestational diabetes compared to nonobese women. Historically, black women are at risk for diabetes. Obesity studies of the
U.S. population show that women are generally fatter than men,
and black women are fatter than white women. Predictably, black
women also have the highest prevalence of diabetes. The risk factor
is likely the obesity rather than gender or race.

Inactivity

Like obesity, inactivity seems to be related to the development of
type II—but not type I—diabetes. Researchers believe that inactivity reduces glucose tolerance, and exercise prevents diabetes secondarily by diminishing the likelihood that one will become
obese.[c]

Environmental Factors

Type I juvenile-onset diabetics are eight times more likely to show
antibodies to pancreatic islet cells than comparison groups of their
nondiabetic parents and siblings.[d] This finding suggests to
researchers that juvenile-onset diabetes may be caused by a virus or
some environmental sensitizing agent that triggers those genetical-
ly susceptible persons to exhibit an autoimmune response of this
sort. As yet, the identity of such an environmental factor is
unknown.

MORTALITY

In 1984, diabetes ranked as the seventh leading cause of death and
took an estimated 35,804 lives. The official mortality statistics for
diabetes deaths are shown in Table 4–4. These figures are thought

---

[a]Baird JD: Is obesity a factor in the aetiology of noninsulin dependent diabetes? In Kobberling
J, Tattersall R, (eds): Serono Symposium No 47 *The Genetics of Diabetes Mellitus.* New
York: Academic, 231–241, 1982
[b]Kempner W, Newborg BC, Peschel RL et al: Treatment of massive obesity with rice/
reduction diet program: An analysis of 106 patients with at least a 45 kg weight loss. *Arch
Int Med* 135: 1575–1584, 1975
[c]Lipman RL, Schnure JJ, Bradley EM et al: Impairment of peripheral glucose utilization in
normal subjects by prolonged bed rest. *J Lab Clin Med* 81:221–223, 1970
[d]Cudworth AG, Spencer KM Gorsuch AN et al: Immunogenetic heterogeneity in insulin-
dependent diabetics. In Kobberling J, Tattersall R (eds): Serono Symposium No. 47, *The
Genetics of Diabetes Mellitus.* New York: Academic, 63–78, 1982.

TABLE 4–4.   Age-specific Death Rates per 100,000 Population for Diabetes Mellitus: United States, 1950–1983

	TOTAL	AGE (IN YEARS)										
		0–1	1–4	5–14	15–24	25–34	35–44	45–54	55–64	65–74	75–84	85+
1983	15.2*	—	0.1	0.1	0.2	1.5	4.0	8.1	24.8	64.6	124.8	195.0
1982	14.4	0.8	0.1	0.1	1.3	1.3	3.1	9.1	25.1	56.1	124.8	194.0
1974	17.7	0.5	0.1	0.2	0.5	1.9	4.3	11.4	31.7	81.6	172.0	248.4
1973	18.2	0.5	0.1	0.2	0.6	2.0	4.6	11.8	34.1	85.4	179.7	245.9
1972	18.6	0.6	0.2	0.2	0.6	2.4	4.9	12.3	33.8	89.7	181.5	255.3
1971	18.6	0.3	0.1	0.3	0.6	2.3	5.1	12.4	35.2	89.5	182.4	248.0
1970	18.9	0.3	0.2	0.2	0.7	2.2	5.3	12.8	36.7	92.1	186.8	230.2
1969	19.1	0.3	0.1	0.2	0.7	2.5	5.4	13.1	37.1	96.7	185.9	262.0
1968	19.2	0.5	0.1	0.2	0.7	2.6	5.3	13.0	39.2	99.5	183.3	258.3
1967	17.7	0.4	0.1	0.3	0.7	2.5	4.8	12.3	36.2	94.2	169.4	234.8
1966	17.7	0.5	0.2	0.3	0.7	2.6	5.0	12.1	35.7	95.7	171.5	234.4
1965	17.1	0.5	0.2	0.3	0.7	2.6	4.7	11.9	36.1	92.6	166.4	220.0
1964	16.9	0.6	0.2	0.3	0.8	2.6	4.8	12.0	37.3	91.4	161.6	204.9
1963	17.2	0.4	0.2	0.3	0.9	2.6	5.0	12.1	37.5	95.1	165.9	206.6
1962	16.8	0.6	0.2	0.3	0.8	2.5	4.6	11.7	36.9	94.0	160.2	206.7
1961	16.4	0.3	0.2	0.3	0.7	2.7	4.7	11.3	35.9	91.4	162.9	184.2
1960	16.7	0.4	0.3	0.4	0.9	2.3	4.5	12.1	37.9	93.4	163.7	181.7
1959	15.9	0.3	0.2	0.4	0.9	2.6	3.8	11.4	37.5	89.9	154.5	158.8
1958	15.9	0.3	0.3	0.3	0.9	2.5	4.1	11.2	37.0	91.6	151.7	169.9
1957	16.0	0.3	0.3	0.4	1.2	2.6	4.5	11.2	38.0	92.5	149.8	158.1
1956	15.7	0.5	0.2	0.3	1.0	2.4	3.8	11.0	37.5	92.1	151.7	162.6
1955	15.5	0.6	0.3	0.4	1.0	2.4	3.9	10.9	37.3	91.7	150.6	163.1
1954	15.6	0.5	0.3	0.4	1.0	2.2	3.9	11.3	38.3	92.3	153.9	155.3
1953	16.3	0.5	0.3	0.4	1.2	2.4	4.1	11.7	41.7	96.2	161.7	156.4
1952	16.4	0.8	0.5	0.6	1.3	2.3	4.0	12.3	40.8	99.7	161.5	152.8
1951	16.3	0.4	0.4	0.5	1.2	2.2	3.9	12.4	42.7	99.8	161.2	151.1
1950	16.2	0.7	0.3	0.6	1.1	2.2	4.2	12.4	42.1	101.2	166.7	150.3

*Not age-adjusted

Source: Advance Report Final Mortality Statistics, 1974
National Center for Health Statistics. Data from the national vital statistics system
Monthly Vital Statistics Report. Vol. 24, No. 11, DHEW Publication No. (HRA) 76–1120
Report of the National Commission on Diabetes Vol. III., Part I, DHEW Publication No. (NIH) 76–102

to considerably underestimate the actual number of deaths. Diabetes is not listed as cause of death on the certificate of an estimated 10% of diagnosed diabetics, especially older ones who usually suffer from several chronic or life-threatening conditions. Many diabetic deaths are attributed to vascular disease, which often results from diabetes. In such instances, vascular disease is really a secondary cause of death.

The U.S. diabetic death rate by age from 1950 to 1983 is shown in Table 4–4.

Figure 4–1 shows the relative differences in diabetes mortality according to sex and race. As is readily apparent, non-whites have a higher diabetes mortality rate than whites. This is especially true of non-white females. White females, on the other hand, have shown a steady decrease in their death rate, making them the lowest risk group (as of 1975).

The diabetes mortality rate in various countries by latest reported year is presented in Table 4–5.

FIG. 4–1. Age-adjusted death rates for diabetes mellitus by color and sex: United States 1950–74

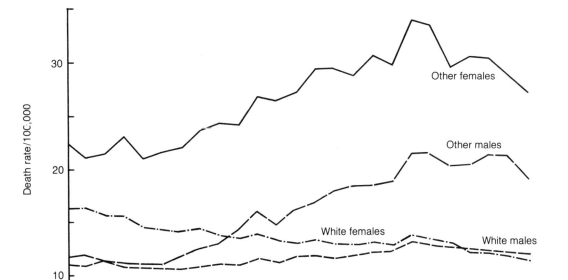

Source: *Report of the National Commission on Diabetes*, Vol. III, Part 1, DHEW Publication No. (NIH) 76–1021

TABLE 4–5. Mortality Rate for Diabetes in Several Countries by Latest Reported Year

COUNTRY	RATE/100,000	YEAR
Costa Rica	9.1	1981
Guatemala	5.0	1980
Chile	12.4	1980
Israel	5.0	1980
Japan	7.3	1980
Kuwait	5.0	1979
Austria	17.0	1981
Bulgaria	12.8	1981
France	13.1	1980
Greece	30.8	1981
Hungary	19.0	1980
Poland	12.6	1980
United Kingdom, England, Wales	9.3	1981
Australia	11.1	1980
United States*	9.6	1982

*National Center for Health Statistics
Source: *U.N. Demographic Yearbook, 1982*

DIABETIC COMPLICATIONS

The mortality rate of diabetics is higher than for the general population. The younger a person is at onset, such as those with juvenile-onset type I diabetes, the higher the mortality. Life expectancy for diabetics is often quoted as one-third the expectancy of the nondiabetic population. An 11-fold excess mortality for juvenile-onset diabetes was determined from one study of insurance company records while a two- to three-fold excess was reported for those who developed diabetes after age 40.[e]

Type I diabetics of short duration often die from diabetic coma. Longer duration type I diabetics, who have not succumbed early on to coma, show diabetic nephropathy as a primary cause of death. Type II diabetics also suffer from renal disease 23 times more often than those of the same age in the general population.[f] Even cardiovascular complications, which are less common in type I than type II diabetics, are nevertheless 11 times more common in type I diabetics than in the general population. Cardiovascular complications are the pre-eminent cause of death in type II diabetics.

[e]Goodkin G: Mortality factors in diabetes, *J Occup Med* 17:716–721, 1975
[f]Geiss LS Herman WH, Teutsch SM et al: Diabetes and renal mortality in the United States (submitted for publication)

Older male type II diabetics are more likely than others to develop peripheral vascular disease. This complication is also closely associated with obesity and cigarette smoking and somewhat associated with hypertension, hyperlipidemia, hyperglycemia and failure to manage the disease.

Complications that cause death sometimes obscure the underlying diabetic cause of death. These complications are the chief reasons why diabetes is a debilitating and often fatal disease. The most serious complications include diabetic coma, stroke, cardiovascular disease, and renal disease. A study of life insurance records from 1951 to 1971 revealed the pattern of diabetic, complication- related death. By far, cardiovascular–renal complications led to the greatest loss of life among diabetics.

CORONARY HEART DISEASE

Studies have surveyed the prevalence of coronary heart disease in groups of living diabetic patients and in the general population. The results of some of these studies listed indicate that black diabetics studied in Nashville and diabetic women adults studied in Cleveland had much higher rates of coronary heart disease (CHD) compared with adults in the general population as were studied in the Framingham Study (Table 4–6).[g] Their rate was also higher than that of a general adult diabetic population, including males studied in 1970. But rates of black and adult female diabetics were lower than the rate of a male and female diabetic population, which included juvenile-onset diabetics as well as adults. The latter group studied in Cleveland in 1955 had a CHD rate of 42%.[h] Generally, studies have determined a frequency of CHD disease among diabetics of 9.5% to 42%; estimates have been given that about 25% of all diabetics suffer from CHD.

Non-CHD diabetics at the beginning of the Framingham Study were monitored for 16 years. At that time, 17% of the 239 diabetics originally free of CHD were symptomatic. Only 9% of the nondiabetic population showed signs of new CHD.

GANGRENE AND AMPUTATION

Because of their greater tendency to develop peripheral vascular disease as well as CHD, gangrene and amputation of toes and legs are not uncommon problems of diabetics. This is particularly true

---

[g]Garcia MJ McNamara PM, Gordon T et al: Morbidity and mortality in diabetes in the Framingham population. *Diabetes* 23:105, 1974
[h]Liebow IM Hellerstein HK, Miller M et al: Arteriosclerotic heart disease in diabetes mellitus: a clinical study of 383 patients. *Amer J Med* 18: 438, 1955

TABLE 4–6.   Reports of Prevalences of Coronary Heart Disease in Groups of Living Diabetic Patients and in General Populations

LOCATION	PATIENT POPULATION	ABNORMALITY	AGE (YEARS)	NUMBER	PERCENTAGE
Cleveland 1955	General diabetic	CHD	10–90	383	42
		MI			6.8
		AP			10
Boston 1957	Adult Diabetic	CHD	40+	288	26
		MI			11
		AP			12
Nashville 1961	Black diabetic	CHD	23–88	100	33
Cleveland 1964	Adult diabetic women	CHD	40–70	58	33
United States 1965	Juvenile diabetic	HD	15+	442	5.4
United States 1970*	Adult diabetic	CHD	20–79	1006	9.5
Rochester, MN* 1976	Adult diabetic	CHD	30+	1028	20
Framingham, MA 1961	General population	CHD	30–62	5209	1.6
Tecumseh, MI 1965	General population	CHD	16–70+	5129	4.1

*CHD at time of diabetes diagnosis
Key: CHD, coronary heart disease; MI, myocardial infarction; AP, angina pectoris; HD, heart disease
Source: *National Diabetes Data Group, 1977*

of mature-onset diabetics who suffer a loss of circulation in their peripheral vessels. Juvenile-onset diabetics tend to experience calcium deposition in these vessels without circulatory impairment.

Gangrene is 20 times more common in the diabetic than it is in the general population. It is reported in 13% to 29% of diabetics at autopsy examination. Results of various studies reveal occlusive peripheral disease in 16% to 58% of living diabetics. In incidence studies, the percentage of diabetics developing this problem within 7 years ranged from 11.3 to 16. Juvenile-onset diabetics, who have the disease for 20 years, show nonocclusive calcium deposition at a rate of 85%.

The results found in several studies dealing with the prevalence of peripheral vascular disease in diabetics are summarized in Table 4–7.

KETOACIDOSIS

Another sometimes-fatal complication, especially in the juvenile-onset type, is diabetic ketoacidosis. Surveys conducted at 15 U.S. hospital centers determined that (1) ketoacidosis-caused deaths ranged from 0.7% to 19% and (2) ketoacidosis accounted for rough-

TABLE 4–7.   Reports of Prevalences of Peripheral Vascular Disease in Diabetes

LOCATION	PATIENT POPULATION	ABNORMALITY	AGE (YEARS)	NUMBER	PERCENTAGE
Minneapolis 1952	Diabetic autopsy	Gangrene	30–91	1,470	13
New Jersey 1953	General diabetic	Physical signs, X-ray calcification	17–64	264	58
Boston 1956	Juvenile diabetic	X-ray calcification	20–49	835	85
Boston 1957	General diabetic	Claudication	10–80	394	16
Philadelphia 1958	General diabetic	Calcification signs and tests	19–80	1,600	54
Boston 1960	Diabetic autopsy	Gangrene		1,854	29
United States 1970	Adult diabetic*	X-ray calcification	20–79	997	16
Rochester, MN 1976	Adult diabetic†	Signs	30+	1,028	8.4

*At diagnosis of diabetes, right lower limb
†At diagnosis of diabetes
Source: *Diabetes Data Group, 1977*

ly 10% of all deaths of diabetics. The mortality due to hyperglycemic coma and lactic acidosis—two other diabetic-related metabolic disorders discovered in the 1970s—ranged from 8% to 23% and from 19% to 33%, respectively.

RENAL DISEASE

Data were gathered from studies of renal disease complications in diabetics. They account for about 50% of deaths in long-term juvenile diabetics and about 6% of deaths in type II diabetics. Dialysis and renal transplant have extended life for diabetics. The prevalence of renal disease in older, living diabetics is in the range of 5% to 51%. Kidney lesions that occur commonly in diabetics are small, vessel-wall abnormalities, diabetic glomerulosclerosis, and arteriolar sclerosis.

Studies of juvenile-onset diabetics in Cincinnati showed albuminuria in 63% of those who had the disease for 35 to 39 years. Proteinuria was found in 38% of diabetics ill for 25 years.[i] A Boston study of a similar group showed a 41% rate.[j] After 5 years of proteinuria, one-half the juvenile-onset diabetics in another Cincinnati study developed renal failure. They had a life expectancy of only 3 years after the onset of renal failure.[k] Estimates provided by several studies are shown in Tables 4–8 and 4–9.

[i]Knowles HC: Long-term juvenile diabetes, treated with unmeasured diet. *Trans Assoc Amer Phys* 84:95, 1971
[j]White P: Natural course and prognosis of juvenile diabetes. *Diabetes* 5:445, 1956
[k]Knowles HC: Magnitude of the renal failure problem in diabetic patients. *Kidney International* 6(4), Suppl 1, New York: Springer-Verlag, 1974

TABLE 4–8.   Prevalences of Albuminuria At Known Duration of Juvenile-Onset Diabetes Mellitus

DURATION OF DIABETES (YEARS)	ALBUMINURIA (%)
5–9	2
15–19	18
25–29	39
35–39	63

Source: *Diabetes Data Group 1977*

TABLE 4–9.   Mortality in Diabetic Patients with Proteinuria

	MORTALITY % AT YEAR	
GROUPS	5	10
Diabetic patients with proteinuria	35	72
Diabetic patients without proteinuria	27	54
Natural expected	17	38

Source: *Diabetes Data Group, 1977*

VISUAL IMPAIRMENT

Visual impairment and blindness are also more common among diabetics. Sight loss often results from neovascularization or new vessel formation. These developments can lead to hemorrhage, scarring, and visual loss. Blindness is 25 times more common in diabetics than in nondiabetics, and at least 5,000 diabetics become blind yearly. The reported prevalence of retinopathy among various diabetic study groups including juvenile and adult types is given in Table 4–10.

The percentage of those with neovascularization has been as high as 59% in studies of juvenile diabetics with a known duration

TABLE 4–10.   Five-Year Visual Deterioration from Retinopathy in Diabetic Patients with Retinopathy

AGE AT DIAGNOSIS (YEAR)	NUMBER	IMPAIRMENT OF VISION (%)	BLIND (%)
0–29	40	3.2	2.8
30–59	81	14.0	3.3
60+	14	32.0	20.0

Source: *Diabetes Data Group, 1977*

of diabetes >30 years as is shown in Table 4–11. In general diabetic populations the rate was as high as 20%.

The prevalences of retinopathy is presented in Table 4–12. The risk is proportional to the time one has been diabetic.

Cataracts in juvenile-onset diabetes are different from those that develop in the general population and adult-onset diabetics. Progression of the cataract is faster, and prevalence in juvenile-onset diabetics has been detected at anywhere from 5% to 47% in different studies. These rates exceed those of nondiabetic young people (Table 4–13).

NEUROPATHY

Another complication of diabetes is neuropathy, a dysfunction of peripheral nerve pathways. The affected nerves may be motor, sen-

TABLE 4–11.   Reported Prevalences of Neovascularization

SOURCE	PATIENT POPULATION	DURATION OF KNOWN DIABETES (YEARS)	NUMBER	PERCENTAGE
Boston 1956	Juvenile diabetic	0–9	879	0
		15–19		18
		25–29		46
		30–34		59
Cincinnati 1971	Juvenile diabetic	20	167	27
		25		40
		30		46
United States 1976	Adult diabetic	6.5*	602	0.7†
Oxford, England 1968	Age at diagnosis <30	0–29		0–14
	Age at diagnosis 30–59	0–29		1–10

*Median duration of known diabetes.
†Right central fundus photo.
Source: *Diabetes Data Group, 1977*

TABLE 4–12.   Reported Prevalences of Retinopathy

SOURCE	PATIENT POPULATION	DURATION OF KNOWN DIABETES (YEARS)	NUMBER	PERCENTAGE
Boston 1956	Juvenile diabetic	20 yrs	879	59
Cincinnati 1971	Juvenile diabetic	20 yrs	167	45
Boston 1957	General diabetic	All durations	370	38
Oxford, England 1968	General diabetic	All durations	2,184*	38
United States 1970	Adult diabetic†	<1 yr	716	16

*3,907 observations on 2,184 patients
†Right central fundus photo; retinopathy includes capillary, venous and arterial pathology excluding exudates
Source: *Diabetes Data Group, 1977*

TABLE 4–13. Frequency of Lens Opacities and Cataracts in 2,820 Observations in 1,827
Diabetics in Relation to Age and Sex

AGE (YEAR)	MALE (%)	FEMALE (%)
0–19	5	0
20–29	5	9
30–39	4	14
40–49	9	29
50–59	32	53
60–69	55	73
70–79	80	84
80+	86	88

Source: *Diabetes Data Group, 1977*

sory, somatic, or autonomic, resulting in leg pain, muscle weakness, abnormalities of stomach, intestinal motility, poor bladder muscle tone, impotence, and dizziness on standing.

A key clinical finding is absence of the ankle jerk on physical examination. Neuropathy, while not fatal, is often incapacitating in longstanding juvenile-onset diabetics. Over 200,000 diabetics suffer from neuropathic disorders in the United States according to the composite estimate gleaned from several studies. The prevalence of this complication varies greatly from study to study in part, however, because investigators use different means to measure neuropathy. The mode of measurement and the prevalence reported by studies conducted from the early 1950s through 1977 are presented in Table 4–14.

DIABETES AND HEALTH RESOURCES

Information on limitation of activity and restricted activity including number of days confined to bed was obtained in the National Health Interview Surveys 1979–1981. Fifty-six percent of all diabetics reported some limitation of activity. On average diabetics experienced 6.4 days in bed annually (Table 4–15).

According to the National Ambulatory Care Survey of 1980, approximately 1.6% of all office visits made that year were primarily because of diabetes; another 2.82% involved a diagnosis of diabetes. This amounted to about 9.5 million visits. The chief reason for office visits was chronic problem flare-ups. Patients older than age 65 years averaged 2.18 drug mentions per visit compared to 1.71 for those 45 to 64 years (Table 4–16).

The distribution of drug mentions by drug category is presented in Table 4–17. Approximately 83% of drugs used were in four basic

TABLE 4–14. Reported Prevalences of Symptoms and Signs of Neuropathy in Diabetes

SOURCE	MEASUREMENT	PATIENTS	NEUROPATHY (%)
Cleveland 1953	Subjective complaints	261	62
Salford, England 1953	General findings	100	57
Brussels 1965	Objective signs	1,175	21
Stockholm 1950	Objective signs	150	49
Rochester, MN 1961	Electromyography, objective signs	103	42
Philadelphia 1958	Impotence	198	55
New York 1952	Skin vessel dilatation	16	44
London 1960	Abnormal Valsalva maneuver	337	20
Toronto 1961	Objective signs	100*	52
Cincinnati 1965	General signs	77*	35
Chicago 1966	Objective signs, motor conduction velocity	107†	10
Aarhus, Denmark 1968	Motor conduction velocity	14‡	100
London 1971	Motor conduction velocity	39‡	100
Edinburgh 1977	Motor conduction velocity, autonomic vascular tests	10‡	100

*Juvenile diabetes
†Juvenile diabetes below age 17
‡Untreated diabetes
Source: *Diabetes Data Group,* 1977

categories, which included cardiovascular drugs, central nervous system drugs, electrolytes, calories and water balance drugs, hormones or synthetic insulin substitutes. The latter were the most commonly mentioned at 40% of all drug mentions followed by cardiovascular drugs at 19%. Again more of these two kinds of drugs were mentioned for older age people as shown in Table 4–17.

As shown in Table 4–18 insulin was mentioned 3.2 million times, its synthetic substitutes, Diabinase, 1.7 million; Orinase, 0.8 million; and Tolinase 0.6 million. Aldomet, Digoxin, and Lanoxin were prominent cardiovascular drugs. The leading diuretics were Lasix and Dyazide. Seventy-two percent of younger patients were treated only with an antidiuretic agent, while older patients required drugs for hypertension and cardiovascular disease. The form in which drugs are used for treating diabetics is shown in Table 4–19.

Exogenous insulin accounted for 18% of all drug mentions while Diabinase, Orinase, and Tolinase—the oral hypoglycemics—accounted for another 18% of the total. The route of administration for people of different ages and sex is presented in Table 4–20. Diabetics were also hospitalized at a rate 2.3 times that of the general population. The number of patient discharges, their rate, and the average length of stay are presented in Table 4–21.

Figure 4–2 shows the differing rates and their trend since 1965 in hospitalization of diabetics age 45 to 64 years. The pattern of increase is unambiguous.

The hospitalization rate by region is presented in Table 4–22. The rate of hospitalization is highest in the north central region but the length of stay is longest in the Northeast.

Diabetics younger than age 65 years dying in 1981 lost an estimated 105,960 years of potential life. This does not include deaths related to diabetes that are not counted as death due to diabetes. The direct costs due to office visits, hospitalizations, and nursing-home care are estimated at $7.9 billion. The annual indirect costs of diabetes including years of life lost are estimated to be about $10 billion. These costs will be incurred until the cause of this disease can be determined and more effective control and preventive measures devised.

FIG. 4–2. Rates per 1,000 population for patients aged 45 to 64 years discharged from short-stay hospitals with a diagnosis of diabetes mellitus, by sex: United States, 1965, 1970, 1975, 1980

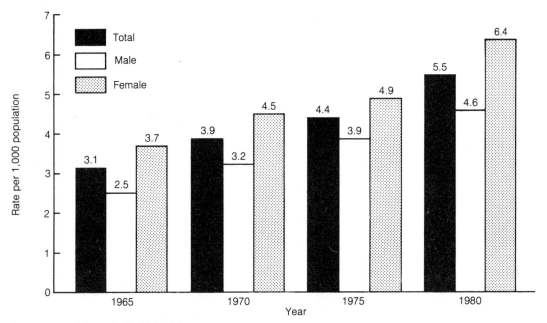

Source: *National Center for Health Statistics*

TABLE 4–15. Impact of Known Diabetes by Age and Selected Health Status Indicators: United States, 1979–81 (data are based on annual one-third subsamples of National Health Interview Survey household interviews of the civilian noninstitutionalized population)

			PERSONS WITH KNOWN DIABETES						
				17 Years and Over					
							65 years and over		
INDICATOR	All Ages	Under 17 Years	All Persons 17 Years and Over	17–44 Years	45–64 Years	All Persons 65 Years and Over	65–74 Years	75 Years and Over
Disability status					Percent			
Persons with limitation of activity due to one or more chronic conditions or impairments	56.0	30.7	56.2	35.6	55.3	65.7	62.4	70.9
Persons for whom diabetes is a cause of limitation of activity	30.5	21.6	30.6	24.7	31.5	32.0	33.2	30.0
Persons with one bed day or more in the past year for diabetes	12.7	43.2	12.4	17.8	12.0	10.8	11.9	9.0
Disability days					Number			
Restricted activity days due to diabetes per person per year	20.8	18.7	20.8	15.4	19.7	24.2	28.0	17.7

Bed days due to diabetes per person per year	6.4	14.1	6.4	4.3	6.2	7.4	5.7	10.3
Bed days due to diabetes per person having 1 bed day or more in the past year for diabetes	41.2	26.7	41.7	18.1	37.4	62.7	39.8	114.0
Work-loss days due to diabetes per currently employed person with diabetes per year	3.1	...	3.1	3.2	3.6	0.6	0.7	...
Medical care				Percent				
Persons who have ever seen a physician for diabetes	99.7	100.0	99.7	99.6	99.7	99.7	99.8	99.5
Persons with 1 or more physician visits in the past year for diabetes	87.0	93.2	87.0	85.0	87.0	87.8	87.7	88.1
Persons ever hospitalized for diabetes	34.6	77.6	34.2	48.8	33.3	29.4	30.0	28.5
Persons taking medicine or treatment recommended by their physician for diabetes	76.1	73.7	76.2	65.5	75.1	81.5	83.1	79.0
Perceived impact								
Persons bothered all the time by diabetes	19.7	19.2	19.7	14.3	20.7	20.8	21.4	19.7
Persons bothered a great deal by diabetes	14.5	8.8	14.7	16.3	15.5	12.8	13.3	11.9
Persons bothered a great deal by diabetes all the time	6.6	4.0	6.7	5.0	6.8	7.2	7.9	6.0
Persons reported to be in fair or poor health	50.8	20.2	51.0	38.8	55.7	50.7	52.9	46.9

Source: *National Center for Health Statistics*. Computed by the Division of Epidemiology and Health Promotion from 1979–81. National Health Interview Survey data provided by the Division of Health Interview Statistics

TABLE 4–16.   Office Visits for Diabetes Mellitus, Number and Percentage of Drug Visits, Number of Drug Mentions, Drug Mention Rate, and Drug Intensity Rate, by Selected Characteristics: United States, 1980

| SELECTED CHARACTERISTICS | OFFICE VISITS | | | Drug Mentions | Drug Mention Rate† | Drug Intensity Rate‡ |
| | All Visits | Drug Visits* | | | Rate per visit | |
	Number in thousands	Number in thousands	Percent	Number in thousands		
Sex						
Both sexes	9,551**	7,592	79.5	17,496	1.83	2.30
Female	5,683	4,544	80.0	11,100	1.95	2.44
Male	3,868	3,048	78.8	6,396	1.65	2.10
Age						
Under 45 years	1,473	1,019	69.2	1,817	1.23	1.78
45–64 years	4,108	3,138	76.4	7,030	1.71	2.24
65 years and over	3,971	3,435	86.5	8,650	2.18	2.52
Race						
White	7,923	6,226	78.6	14,545	1.84	2.34
Black	1,510	1,290	85.4	2,774	1.84	2.15
Problem status						
New problem	871	602	69.2	1,019	1.17	1.69
Old problem	8,680	6,990	80.5	16,477	1.90	2.36
Major reason for visit						
Acute problem	1,087	879	80.9	1,831	1.68	2.08
Chronic problem, routine	7,122	5,660	79.5	12,962	1.82	2.29
Chronic problem, flareup	805	689	85.5	2,034	2.53	2.95
Post surgery/post injury	117¶	39¶	33.6¶	95¶	.81¶	2.44¶
Nonillness care	419	324¶	77.3¶	574¶	1.37¶	1.77¶

*A visit in which one or more drugs were ordered or provided
†Drug mentions divided by number of visits
‡Drug mentions divided by number of drug visits
**Included races other than white and black not shown as separate categories
¶May be unreliable
Source: *Vital and Health Statistics*, Series 13, No. 71

TABLE 4–17. Number and Percentage Distribution, and Rate per 100 Visits of Drug Mentions in Office Visits for Diabetes Mellitus by Therapeutic Category, According to Sex and Age of the Patient: United States, 1980

THERAPEUTIC CATEGORY	BOTH SEXES	SEX		AGE		
		Female	Male	Under 45 Years	45–64 Years	65 Years and Over
			Number of mentions in thousands			
All therapeutic categories	17,496	11,100	6,396	1,817	7,030	8,650
			Percent distribution			
Total	100.0	100.0	100.0	100.0	100.0	100.0
Cardiovascular drugs	18.5	17.8	19.8	6.0*	17.9	21.7
Central nervous system drugs	9.4	9.7	8.9*	8.8*	8.5*	10.2
Electrolytic, caloric, and water balance	14.8	15.5	13.6	6.7*	15.4	16.1
Hormones and synthetic substitutes	39.8	38.0	42.8	57.9	38.3	37.2
All other therapeutic categories	17.5	19.0	14.9	20.6	19.9	14.8
			Drug mention rate per 100 visits			
Cardiovascular drugs	34	35	33	7*	31	47
Central nervous system drugs	17	19	15	11*	15*	22
Electrolytic, caloric, and water balance	27	30	23	8*	26	35
Hormones and synthetic substitutes	73	74	71	71	66	81

*Based on the classification system of the American Hospital Formulary Service.
†May be unreliable
Source: *Vital and Health Statistics*, Series 13, No. 71

TABLE 4–18.   Number and Percentage Distribution of Drug Mentions in Office Visits for Diabetes Mellitus by Most Frequently Mentioned Specific Drugs Described by Principal Generic Ingredient(s) and Principal Therapeutic Category: United States, 1980

NAME OF DRUG	DRUG MENTIONS		PRINCIPAL GENERIC INGREDIENT(S)†	PRINCIPAL THERAPEUTIC CATEGORY‡
	Number in thousands	Percent distribution		
All drugs	17,496	100.0	. . .	. . .
Insulin	3,192	18.2	Insulin	Insulin and anti-diabetic agents
Diabinese	1,728	9.9	Chlorpropamide	Insulin and anti-diabetic agents
Orinase	792	4.5	Tolbutamide	Insulin and anti-diabetic agents
Tolinase	621	3.5	Tolazamide	Insulin and anti-diabetic agents
Lasix	621	3.5	Furosemide	Diuretics
Dyazide	491	2.8	Triamterene, hydrochlorothiazide	Diuretics
Aldomet	479	2.7	Methyldopa	Hypotensive agents
Lanoxin	391**	2.2**	Digoxin	Cardiac drugs
Digoxin	322**	1.8**	Digoxin	Cardiac drugs
Residual	8,858	50.6	—	—

*Based on the physician's entry on the Patient Record form; entry may be a brand or generic name
†If only one generic ingredient is listed, the physician's entry is the generic drug or a brand name drug that consists chiefly of a single generic ingredient; may not include all ingredients for every combination drug
‡Based on the classification system of the American Hospital Formulary Service
**May be unreliable
Source: Vital and Health Statistics, Series 13, No. 71

TABLE 4–19.   Number and Percentage Distribution of Drugs Used in Office Visits for Diabetes Mellitus by Form of Use, According to Most Frequently Used Generic Substances: United States, 1980

GENERIC SUBSTANCE	DRUGS USED	Form of Use		
		Total	Single Ingredient	Combinations
	Number in thousands	Percentage distribution		
Chlorpropamide	1,733	100.0	100.0	—
Digoxin	714	100.0	100.0	—
Furosemide	626	100.0	100.0	—
Hydrochlorothiazide	1,331	100.0	33.7	66.3
Insulin	3,198	100.0	100.0	—
Methyldopa	617	100.0	83.7	16.3
Tolazamide	621	100.0	100.0	—
Tolbutamide	820	100.0	100.0	—
Triamterene	491	100.0	—	100.0

Source: *Vital and Health Statistics,* Series 13, No. 71

TABLE 4–20.   Number and Percentage Distribution of Selected Antidiabetic Agents Mentioned in Office Visits for Diabetes Mellitus by Route of Administration of the Drug, According to Sex and Age of the Patient: United States, 1980

SEX AND AGE	Number of Selected Antidiabetic Agents in Thousands	Total	Oral*	Injection[†]
Sex		Percentage distribution		
Female	3,740	100.0	51.2	48.8
Male	2,593	100.0	47.2	52.8
Age				
25–44 years	716	100.0	21.9	78.1
45–64 years	2,476	100.0	48.8	51.2
65 years and over	2,873	100.0	60.5	39.5

*Diabinese (chlorpropamide), Orinase (tolbutamide), and Tolinase (tolazamide)
[†]Insulin
Source: *Vital and Health Statistics,* Series 13, No. 71

TABLE 4–21.   Number and Rate of Hospital Discharges and Average Length of Stay, United States, 1980

PREVALENCE	BOTH SEXES	MALE	FEMALE
Number in Thousands	645	245	400
Rate per 1000	2.9	2.3	3.5
Average Length of Stay	10.5	10.1	10.7

Source: *National Hospital Discharge Survey, 1980*

TABLE 4–22.   Hospitalization Rate and Average Length of Stay, United States, 1980, of Diabetics

LOCALE	RATE PER 1,000	AVERAGE LENGTH OF STAY
All Regions	2.9	10.5
Northeast	3.1	12.9
North Central	3.2	10.3
South	3.1	9.8
West	1.8	8.1

Source: *National Hospital Discharge Survey, 1980*

Renal
Disease   5

Diabetes can seriously reduce renal function (see Chapter 4). Since the kidneys play a major role in metabolism, hormone production, the function of several other organs, the homeostasis of body fluid, and the excretion of waste, renal disease or dysfunction related to diabetes or to any of several other ailments requires medical evaluation and treatment.

THE KIDNEY

The kidneys in the average adult filter about 5 quarts of body fluid every 45 minutes. Much of the fluid is reabsorbed; 1.5 quarts are excreted daily with waste material, such as urea—a breakdown product of protein. The kidneys accomplish their work through the filtering activity of 1 to 2 million nephrons. Each nephron consists of small blood vessels and capillaries, comprising the glomerulus encased in a double-walled capsule. The capsules are attached to long-winding tubes of varying length and thickness.

Kidney disease or dysfunction, or both, has many causes. Kidney dysfunction can be caused by a congenital anomaly, such as medullary sponge kidney, a cystic condition that often goes undetected until midlife. Another less benign congenital kidney disease is medullary cystic disease, which leads to complete renal failure and the need for dialysis or transplant by adulthood. Similarly, polycystic kidney disease also progresses to uremia, which is usually fatal.

Kidney disease can also develop after certain infections or because of obstruction, autoimmune reactions, ischemia, or vascular disease. The major classifications of renal disease are listed in the International Classification of Diseases (ICDA) as 580–589; nephritis, nephrotic syndrome, and nephrosis.

NEPHRITIS, NEPHROTIC SYNDROME AND NEPHROSIS, ICDA (580–589)

Illness designated under 580–589 as renal disease (which excludes deaths due to renal infection [590]) is the 13th leading cause of death in the United States. In 1983, an estimated 18,710 deaths were caused by renal disease specified as nephritis, nephrotic syndrome, and nephrosis. This number represented an increase over the 1982 level of 18,102. This was contrary to the general declining trend in renal-related mortality that has occurred since 1950. In 1950, the mortality rate was almost 17 per 100,000; by the 1980s, it was around 8 per 100,000. The estimated number of deaths and the rate of renal mortality is presented in Table 5–1.

ACUTE GLOMERULONEPHRITIS AND NE-PHROTIC SYNDROME, ICDA (580–581)

Acute glomerulonephritis includes proliferative glomerulonephritis, poststreptococcal glomerulonephritis, rapidly progressive glomerulonephritis, and glomerulonephritis induced by diseases, such

TABLE 5–1. Deaths and Death Rate of Nephritis, Nephrotic Syndrome, and Nephrosis, United States 1982–84

YEAR	NUMBER	CRUDE RATE/100,000
1984	20,570	8.7
1983	18,710	8.0
1982:	18,102	7.7
Male	9,165	8.1
Female	8,937	7.5
White	14,453	7.3
Black	3,649	10.8

Source: *Monthly Vital Statistics Reports*, Vol. 33, numbers 9 and 12

as infectious hepatitis, interstitial focal nephritis, and nephropathy.

The term "nephritis" is a general designation for renal inflammatory disease. One of the more common types of inflammation causing acute renal failure is acute poststreptococcal glomerulonephritis. In this disorder, inflammation of the glomeruli follows a streptococcal infection of the respiratory tract or in rare cases, of the skin. Poststreptococcal glomerulonephritis is most common in children and 95% recover. Adults have a 70% recovery rate; the remaining 30% deteriorate to chronic renal failure.

RAPIDLY PROGRESSING GLOMERULONE-PHRITIS, ICDA (580.4)

Rapidly progressing glomerulonephritis is a much less common form of glomerulonephritis than is poststreptococcal glomerulonephritis. The rapidly progressing form occurs as part of a mulitsystem disease, such as systemic lupus erythematosis (SLE) or polyarteritis nodosa in 40% of all cases; 30% involve antibody reaction against the glomerular basal lamina. Some cases also seem to involve immune complex disease. It involves extracapillary proliferation in most glomeruli.

Onset is often concomitant with fatigue, weakness, nausea, vomiting, anorexia, and malaise. One-half of all patients develop edema and are febrile before renal failure occurs. Treatment usually necessitates dialysis. Plasmapheresis is also used when the cause is fulminant immune complex disease. Spontaneous remission is rare when this form of glomerular disease is idiopathic but possible when a controllable disease has precipitated this disorder.

OTHER ACUTE GLOMERULONEPHRITIS SYNDROMES, ICDA (580.–)

Interstitial focal nephritis refers local inflammation in interstitial areas, whereas proliferative glomerulonephritis refers to inflammation and proliferation of glomerular cells. Nephropathy can refer to either sclerotic lesions with inflammatory disease or necrosis of cells.

NEPHROTIC SYNDROME: PRIMARY GLOMERULONEPHRITIS

Nephrotic syndrome develops as a consequence of primary glomerulonephritis. In children, primary glomerulonephritis is often correlated with lipid deposits in the tubules. In adults, the basement membrane of the glomeruli becomes thick, causing inflammation, kidney damage, and eventually renal failure.

. Up to 20% of adults with primary glomerulonephritis suffer from focal glomerulosclerosis that leads to nephrotic syndrome. This form of glomerular disease can develop at any age spontaneously, but it also follows kidney transplantation and heroin use. Focal glomerulosclerosis usually causes hyaline sclerosis.

These primary glomerular diseases causing nephrotic syndrome involve increased protein permeability of the glomeruli with accompanying protein excretion—especially albumin. Nephrotic syndrome can be recognized by severe dependent edema of (1) the ankles, (2) periorbital area of the face or (3) sacrum; consistent proteinuria in excess of 3.5 g daily; and an increase in hyaline and waxy, fatty casts and oval fat bodies in the urine. Diagnosis is confirmed by kidney biopsy examination.

Patients may develop orthostatic hypotension, lethargy, fatigue, anorexia, pallor, and depression. They should be watched for signs of accelerated atherosclerosis, coagulation disorders, thromboembolic vascular occlusion, malnutrition, and infection.

If the cause of nephrotic syndrome can be eliminated—as when glomerulonephritis is caused by heroin or the ingestion of other nephrotoxic substances, such as mercury or gold—treatment is usually successful. Treatment or management of diseases that cause nephrotoxic syndrome can also effect improved kidney function. Such diseases include diabetes, sickle-cell anemia, multiple myeloma, tuberculosis, and congestive heart failure. When nephrotic syndrome is idiopathic, treatment is only supportive, involving adherence to a high-protein, low-sodium diet accompanied by diuretics to reduce edema and by antibiotics to combat infection.

The estimated number of deaths and death rate of acute glomerulonephritis and nephrotic syndrome is summarized in Table 5–2.

TABLE 5–2.   Deaths and Death Rate from Acute Glomerulonephritis and Nephrotic Syndrome, United States, 1982–84

YEAR	NUMBER	CRUDE RATE/100,000
1984	330	0.1
1983	350	0.1
1982:	309	0.1
Males	151	0.1
Females	158	0.1
White	247	0.2
Black	62	0.2

Source: *Monthly Vital Statistics Report*, Vol. 33, numbers 9 and 12

CHRONIC GLOMERULONEPHRITIS, NEPHRITIS AND NEPHROPATHY NOT SPECIFIED AS ACUTE OR CHRONIC, AND RENAL SCLEROSIS, UNSPECIFIED, ICDA (582–3, 587)

CHRONIC GLOMERULONEPHRITIS

Chronic glomerulonephritis, an inflammation of the glomeruli that slowly causes tissue scarring and sclerosis, leads ultimately to complete renal failure. It often exists undetected until tissue damage is extensive, making renal impairment irreversible. It is caused by diseases, such as SLE hemolytic-uremic syndrome, and Goodpasture's syndrome. Chronic glomerulonephritis can also follow poststreptococcal glomerulonephritis, rapidly progressive glomerulonephritis, membranous glomerulopathy, and focal glomerulosclerosis.

It may first become apparent as nephrotic syndrome, or it may accelerate to advanced stage uremic symptoms, including azotemia, nausea, vomiting, pruritus, dyspnea, malaise and fatiguability, edema, anemia, and hypertension. The last-mentioned complication can lead to cardiac hypertrophy and congestive heart failure. When renal failure is advanced, treatment requires dialysis or transplantation. Other treatment involves control of hypertension, fluid balance, edema, and infection.

NEPHRITIS AND NEPHROPATHY NOT SPECIFIED AS ACUTE OR CHRONIC, ICDA (583)

This category includes necrotic lesions of the renal cortex, lesions of renal medullary necrosis and nephritis, and nephropathy not specified as chronic or acute in diseases classified elsewhere, such as diabetes.

The estimated deaths and mortality rate from chronic glomerulonephritis, nephritis, and nephropathy are listed in Table 5–3.

TABLE 5–3.   The Deaths and Death Rate from Chronic Glomerulonephritis, Nephritis, and Nephropathy, United States 1982–84

YEAR	NUMBER	CRUDE RATE/100,000
1984	1,770	0.8
1983	1,810	0.8
1982:	1,946	0.8
Males	984	0.9
Females	962	0.8
White	388	0.8
Black	353	1.3

Source: *Monthly Vital Statistics Report*, Vol. 33, numbers 9 and 12

RENAL FAILURE, DISORDERS RESULTING FROM IMPAIRED RENAL FUNCTION AND SMALL KIDNEY OF UNKNOWN CAUSE, ICDA (584–586, 588–589)

ACUTE RENAL FAILURE AND KIDNEY STONES

Acute renal failure occurs when renal function ceases. It is sudden and usually reversible when treated. If untreated, it may deteriorate to end-stage renal disease (ESRD) leading to death. Acute renal failure is caused by many of the disorders just discussed, including acute poststreptococcal glomerulonephritis, nephrotoxins, acute pyelonephritis, and systemic diseases, such as SLE, polyarteritis nodosa, sickle-cell anemia, and cardiovascular disorders. It can also occur because of decreased bloodflow during shock, hemorrhage, sepsis, ascites, and burns or because of obstruction caused by kidney stones and blood clots.

Renal calculi (kidney stones) form when normally dissolved substances precipitate out of urine as calcium oxalate and calcium phosphate. Stones usually form in the renal pelvis or calyces. Large stones can injure tissue or obstruct urine flow to the bladder.

The chief symptom of kidney stones is pain. Typically, diagnosis is determined through radiographic and kidney ultrasonography. Blood, crystals, pus, casts, and white blood cells (WBCs) may be detected in the urine. Most stones are small and can be passed out of the kidney and bladder through vigorous hydration. Patients are usually given diuretics and substances for pain relief and infection control. They may also be given a low-calcium, high-ascorbic acid diet to prevent formation of additional stones. When stones are larger than 5 cm in diameter, removal may be necessary or attempts may be made to shatter the stones by high-frequency sound waves.

The incidence of kidney stones as reported by hospital discharge records is probably a significant underestimate of their presence in the general population (Table 5–4).

RENAL INFECTIONS

As already discussed, acute renal failure can follow respiratory streptococcal infection. It can also occur because of many other kidney infections. Acute bacterial pyelonephritis or acute infective tubulointerstitial nephritis is often caused by invasion of *Escherichia coli* from the urethral meatus, especially in females in childhood or during pregnancy. Diabetics and those with obstructions like those caused by kidney stones also seem to be more susceptible.

The infection may cause a pattern of patchy inflammation and tissue destruction. Abdominal rigidity may develop as well as a palpable, tender, enlarged kidney. The patient may experience chills, nausea, pain, fever, and urinary symptoms, such as frequent and urgent need to urinate.

Diagnosis is confirmed by urinalysis. Treatment consists of administering antibiotics with urine culture monitoring of the infection. The death rate associated with renal infection is summarized in Table 5–5.

TABLE 5–4. Incidence of Patients Hospitalized with Kidney Calculi, United States 1982

PATIENT STATISTICS	NUMBER	RATE/10,000
All ages	2,970	12.9
15 years old	1,530	14.3
45–64 years old	990	22.2
65 years old	420	15.8
Male	1,960	17.6
Female	1,010	8.5
White	2,570	13.0
Black	180	5.3
Average length of stay (days)	4.8	
Patient discharges:		
Northeast	530	
North Central	780	
South	1,220	
West	430	

Source: *Monthly Vital Statistics Report*, Vol. 33, numbers 9 and 12

TABLE 5–5.   Deaths and Death Rate from Renal Infection, United States, 1982–84

YEARS	NUMBER	CRUDE RATE/100,000
1984	1,850	0.8
1983	1,890	0.8
1982:	2,218	1.0
Males	733	0.7
Female	1,485	1.2
White	1,953	0.8
Black	249	1.3

Source: *Monthly Vital Statistics Report*, Vol. 33 numbers 9 and 12

CHRONIC RENAL FAILURE

Chronic renal failure occurs after most renal function is lost. Those afflicted may be symptomless until 75% of glomerular filtration capacity is lost. The disease deteriorates through several stages of severity—from diminished renal reserve to renal insufficiency to uremia. Nocturia may be the only symptom during the first stage as the patient compensates for reduced renal function. In the last stage, gastrointestinal ulceration, bleeding, and malnutrition are common as is hypertension.

Laboratory findings include nitrogen retention, acidosis, anemia, and elevated urea and creatinine levels. Sometimes the condition can be reversed. Generally, however, it leads to ESRD, which is treatable with dialysis and kidney transplantation.

Patients with various types of renal failure as well as with disorders resulting from impaired renal function and small kidney of unknown cause (ICDA 584–586, 588–587) are profiled in Table 5–6.

TABLE 5–6.   Deaths and Death Rate Associated with Renal Failure and Diseases (ICDA 584–586, 588–589), United States, 1982–84

YEAR	NUMBER	CRUDE RATE/100,000
1984	18,470	7.8
1983	16,550	7.1
1982:	15,847	6.8
Male	8,030	7.1
Female	7,817	6.6
White	12,648	9.5
Black*	3,005	10.9

Source: *Monthly Vital Statistics Report*, Vol. 33, numbers 9 and 12
*Does not include other non-whites

DIALYSIS

Patients with acute kidney failure experience an increase in extra-cellular fluid volume, a buildup of urea, creatinine, and uric acid, metabolic acidosis, and hyperkalemia. As oliguria persists or as uremia develops, dialysis is usually required. Dialysis may also be needed for patients with stable chronic renal failure if the condition is complicated by another illness, or if they show signs of congestive heart failure. Patients with worsening chronic renal failure require dialysis on a permanent basis when their GFR tells below 5 to 8 ml/minute. At this level, patients may develop unremitting nausea and vomiting, encephalopathy, neuropathy, pleuritis, uremia, and pericarditis, conditions that underline the urgency of dialysis. There are three kinds of dialysis.

HEMODIALYSIS

Hemodialysis removes excessive concentrations of waste material, such as nitrogenous products, from blood by diffusing the concentrated solution across a semipermeable membrane. In hemodialysis, blood is circulated from the patient to an artificial kidney machine where it comes into contact with dialysate in a membrane-like unit. Dialysate is a water-concentrate solution that approximates the electrolytic composition of interstitial fluid. It includes glucose, sodium chloride, potassium acetate, calcium, and magnesium. Unwanted blood elements transfer to the dialysate, and the "cleared blood" is returned to the patient. Blood is channeled from the patient by an arteriovenous shunt or fistula. The latter is preferred because it minimizes infections and clotting.

Patients generally report to their dialysis center three times weekly. Each treatment requires 4 to 6 hours, an interval that can be disruptive to normal living schedules of work or school, or both.

PERITONEAL DIALYSIS

Peritoneal dialysis calls for diffusion through the patient's peritoneum instead of a mechanical membrane filtering unit like the one used in hemodialysis. The effect of peritoneal dialysis is similar to that of hemodialysis. Its advantage is that the patient can treat himself in the home setting without special equipment. This is generally cheaper and much more convenient.

Λ sterile plastic catheter is inserted into one of the patient's abdominal gutters. This allows peritoneal irrigation with sterile solutions. Local anesthetic is usually used during catheterization. When the catheter is properly positioned, solution is infused. The stages of dialysis allow for an inflow period, a dwell period, and a gravity drain period—all of them taking less than 1 hour for a 2-liter dialysate. The complete treatment lasts 24 to 72 hours.

CONTINUOUS AMBULATORY PERITONEAL DIALYSIS

Another method of dialysis is continuous ambulatory peritoneal dialysis (CAPD). This process usually involves four 2-liter exchanges daily to control uremia. Because CAPD is continuous, blood can be cleared at much higher levels than the 50% to 60% of hemodialysis and peritoneal dialysis, and patients feel better. However, repeated episodes of peritonitis have been a persistent side effect, together with backache and weight gain. Recent design changes appear to lower the frequency of peritonitis.

Dialysis patients using any of the processes described require intense psychosocial support and medical monitoring. They can develop several mental disorders. They are also vulnerable to hemorrhage because of anticlotting agents, seizures because of osmotic shifts, and suicide because of depression.

END-STAGE RENAL DISEASE PROGRAM

Amendments to the Social Security Act under Medicare, Section 2991 adopted in 1972, extended Medicare coverage to patients with permanent renal failure who require either dialysis or transplantation. To qualify, recipients must also have social security coverage at the onset of their disease and be either a current beneficiary or the dependent of an eligible person.

The 50 states were divided into 32 administrative regions and the ESRD network was established. Each region includes several government-approved treatment facilities. The Health Care Financing Administration (1) administers the program, (2) monitors the quality of care, (3) oversees reimbursement, and (4) collects treatment statistics on both the renal disease population and their health-care providers.

Since its inception, the ESRD program has grown dramatically as the patient base and expenditures have increased (Fig. 5–1).

FIG. 5–1. ESRD program growth

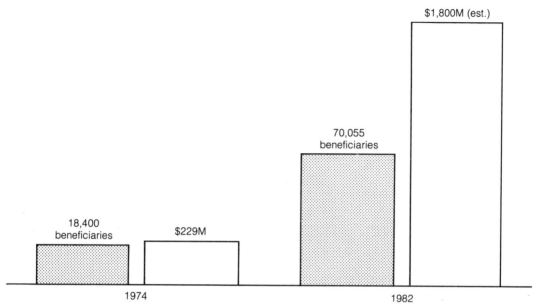

Source: *Medicare Annual Report,* 1982

DIALYSIS FACILITIES

The certified ESRD facilities providing dialysis service have also increased since 1973 (Fig. 5–2). The number shown as of 1982 does not include newly certified facilities or those that provide dialysis on an emergency back-up basis without providing it as a daily routine service. Of the 1,218 facilities approved to provide dialysis and transplantation services as of 1982, 689 were hospital-based with 8 approved only for transplants. Both dialysis and transplantation were provided by 149 hospitals and 532 engaged only in dialysis.

The hospital-based dialysis facilities in the various states correspond with population needs. The most populous or largest states, or both have more than 15 centers; less populated states in the northern mountain area of Montana, Wyoming, and the Dakotas have five or fewer centers (Fig. 5–3).

The independent dialysis facilities in the various states showed a different pattern than did hospital-based facilities. As of 1982, independent dialysis facilities were not always the most numerous in the most populated states. New York, e.g., had fewer than Texas or Alabama (Fig. 5–4).

Just under two-thirds of the dialysis facilities in the ESRD program were nonprofit (Fig. 5–5).

FIG. 5–2. Number of certified ESRD facilities. It includes all ESRD Medicare approved facilities, not just those providing outpatient maintenance dialysis.

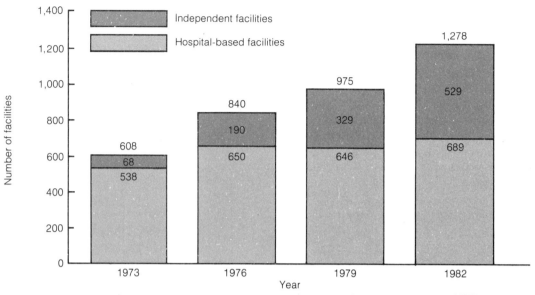

Source: *The National Listing of Providers Furnishing Kidney Dialysis and Transplant Services. January 1983—HCFA*

FIG. 5–3. Dialysis facilities, hospital—1982

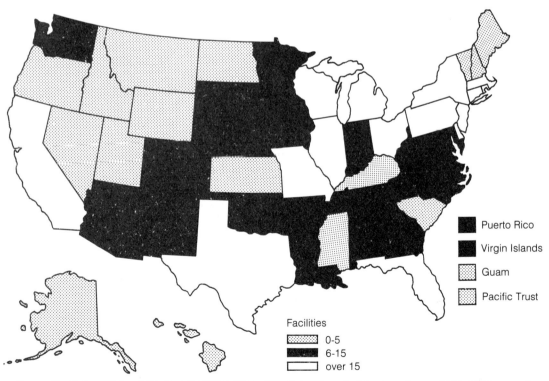

Source: *The National Listing of Providers Furnishing Kidney Dialysis and Transplant Services. January 1983—HCFA*; secondary source: *Annual Medicare Report,* 1982

FIG. 5–4. Dialysis facilities, independent—1982

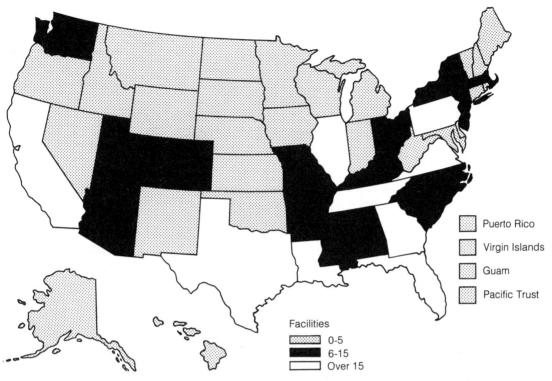

Facilities
- 0-5
- 6-15
- Over 15

Puerto Rico
Virgin Islands
Guam
Pacific Trust

Source: *The National Listing of Providers Furnishing Kidney Dialysis and Transplant Services. January 1983*—HCFA; secondary source: *Annual Medicare Report,* 1982

FIG. 5–5. Type of ownership—profit vs. nonprofit, 1171 ESRD dialysis providers, 1982

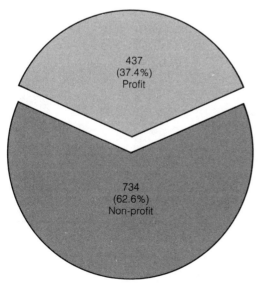

437
(37.4%)
Profit

734
(62.6%)
Non-profit

115

Source: *The National Listing of Providers Furnishing Kidney Dialysis and Transplant Services. January 1983*—HCFA; secondary source: *Annual Medicare Report,* 1982

The distribution of dialysis facilities among for-profit hospitals, free-standing facilities, and hospital satellites vs. nonprofit entities of similar kinds is summarized in Table 5–7. The largest proportion of such facilities were nonprofit hospitals followed by for-profit, freestanding facilities.

The patients receiving dialysis by setting and modality for several recent years are represented in Figure 5–6. The number of total

TABLE 5–7.   Renal Facilities

| | PROFIT | | | NON PROFIT | | |
TOTAL	Hospitals	Free-standing facilities	Hospital satellites	Hospitals	Free-standing facilities	Hospital satellites
1218	14	423	0	643	104	34

*These figures represent the facilities approved to provide maintenance dialysis services to ESRD patients as of December 21, 1982.
Weekly Health Insurance Merge (WHIM) *Record* (HCFA); *ESRD Facility Survey Tables* (BSS, HCFA); *Bureau of Eligibility, Reimbursement and Coverage* (HCFA); *National Listing of Providers Furnishing Kidney Dialysis and Transplant Services (BSS, HCFA);* secondary source: *Annual Medicare Report,* 1982

FIG. 5–6.   Chronic dialysis patients being treated by Medicare certified suppliers of ESRD services in the United States by treatment setting, January 1979–December 1982

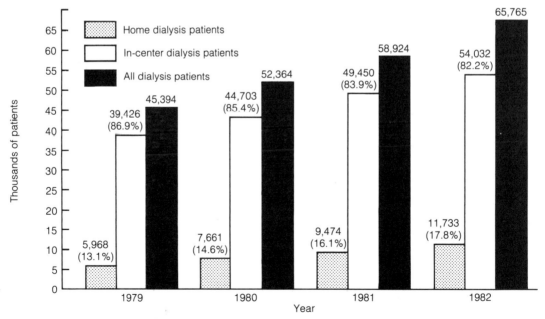

Source: *ESRD Medical Information System 1979, 1980, 1981 and 1982 Facility Surveys;* secondary source: *Annual Medicare Report,* 1982

dialysis patients has been increasing steadily, jumping 11.6% from 58,924 to 65,765 between 1981 and 1982 alone. But the proportion receiving in-center dialysis has declined from 86.9% in 1979 to 82.2% in 1982. By the same token, the proportion of patients receiving cheaper and more convenient home dialysis increased from 13.1% in 1979 to 17.8% by 1982.

The breakdown of patients according to dialysis modality by ESRD regional network is shown in Table 5–8. The patients receiving their dialysis at a facility assisted by staff instead of at home include 51,499 receiving hemodialysis and 874 peridialysis who were assisted by staff. Another 1,071 were self-assisted when undergoing in-unit hemodialysis and peritoneal dialysis. Those training in methods of self-dialysis included another 588, or 1.1%, of all patients, whereas 11,733, or 17.8%, patients underwent dialysis at home.

The percentage of dialysis patients dialysized at home by state in 1982 is shown in Figure 5–7. In general, low population density states had the highest proportion of home dialysis patients, as one might expect where there might be fewer centers, each located farther away from the average patient's home.

The changing proportion of home dialysis patients using hemodialysis, peritoneal, and CAPD between 1979 and 1982 is graphically portrayed in Figure 5–8.

Cost containment and convenience have prompted efforts to increase the number of home-dialysis patients. For similar reasons, patients receiving in-unit treatment are encouraged to become self-care patients. Comparison of the success in achieving self-care status between 1979 and 1982 is shown in Table 5–9. The proportion of self-care home patients plus self-care patients receiving treatment at centers and those being trained in self-care techniques have increased from 15.7% of the total dialysis population to 20.4% of all patients.

MORTALITY

Data have been collected on the survival of dialysis patients according to length of treatment, age, sex, and race (Table 5–10). The total age-adjusted death rate for white males per 1,000 patients was higher at 142.1 than for any other cohort. Overall, nonwhite females seemed to fare best, although they did not survive longer than other groups at young ages, especially those younger than age 20 years.

The longevity of patients calculated by years treated since the study began in 1973 to death, transplant, or 1981, whichever came

TABLE 5–8. Patients Receiving Care As Of 12/31/82

ESRD Network	Facilities Surveyed and Reporting	Total Patients	STAFF ASSISTED DIALYSIS		SELF-DIALYSIS IN-UNIT		SELF-DIALYSIS TRAINING			HOME PATIENTS		
			Hemo-dialysis	Peri-dialysis	Hemo-dialysis	Peri-dialysis	Hemo-dialysis	Peri-dialysis	CAPD*	Hemo-dialysis	Peri-dialysis	CAPD
1	9	435	230	1	120	0	10	1	2	36	11	24
2	27	1,658	925	21	4	0	22	1	11	466	42	166
3	52	2,890	2,357	4	94	0	24	0	6	139	10	256
4	88	4,867	4,306	7	75	0	34	0	9	90	26	320
5	28	1,020	668	5	24	0	2	0	3	199	19	100
6	31	1,101	892	2	8	0	1	0	4	47	3	144
7	27	1,039	804	4	0	0	1	1	3	123	17	86
8	18	775	522	5	0	0	7	1	2	79	27	132
9	31	1,796	1,263	3	0	0	15	0	10	199	16	290
10	32	983	709	25	0	0	3	0	4	81	17	144
11	74	4,673	3,787	21	112	0	37	3	13	199	92	409
12	37	1,384	1,249	18	2	0	1	0	0	27	23	64
13	22	797	489	16	38	0	1	0	6	60	3	184
14	34	2,186	1,535	98	17	0	15	1	4	142	28	346
15	63	3,071	2,607	80	109	0	13	0	8	79	11	164
16	14	1,408	701	4	2	0	17	0	4	286	0	394
17	23	1,294	918	29	33	0	4	0	7	57	0	245
18	65	3,417	2,572	5	7	0	14	1	4	339	89	386
19	71	3,620	3,221	16	6	0	5	0	3	80	25	264
20	53	3,085	2,549	28	65	0	12	0	1	144	31	255
21	20	1,651	1,211	2	0	0	6	1	1	179	63	188
22	47	2,772	2,054	107	21	0	18	1	6	115	39	411
23	23	1,320	1,143	9	15	0	2	0	0	37	0	114
24	59	2,837	2,288	12	57	8	23	4	5	126	57	257
25	65	4,818	4,024	123	30	1	21	0	11	326	7	275
26	24	1,292	893	20	67	0	26	0	4	121	20	136
27	15	875	682	14	16	1	1	0	14	27	3	117
28	37	2,385	1,996	18	9	0	4	1	5	181	28	143
29	15	863	732	37	0	0	0	0	0	57	8	29
30	43	1,962	1,560	23	0	0	16	1	2	129	44	187
31	17	891	652	30	48	1	8	2	3	59	24	64
32	26	2,600	1,955	87	81	0	45	0	6	165	33	228
Total	1,190	65,765	51,499	874	1,060	11	408	19	161	4,394	816	6,523

*CAPD, continuous ambulatory peritoneal dialysis
Source: *ESRD Medical Information System 1982 Facility Surveys;* secondary source: *Annual Medicare Report,* 1982

FIG. 5–7   Home dialysis patients—1982

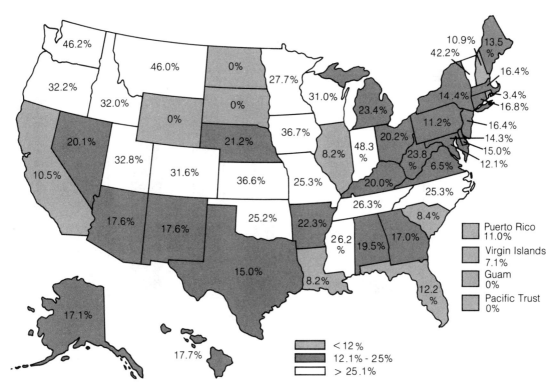

Source: *ESRD Medical Information System 1982 Surveys;* secondary source: *Annual Medicare Report,* 1982

first, is presented in Table 5–11. Clearly, survival within a treatment group improves the longer the group members are in treatment. The weakest patients die earliest. Survival of those 907 patients who were alive at the beginning of the seventh year of treatment was 89%. Only 54 people in this group died during the seventh year. Cumulatively, of course, overall survival by the end of the seventh year of all the patients in the study since 1973 was only 27% crudely measured and 30% when calculated as a relative survival rate.

The major reasons for changes in the number of patients treated by Medicare-certified suppliers of ESRD services between 1979 and 1982 were either receipt of a kidney transplant or death, or both (Fig. 5–9).

FIG. 5–8.   Home patient modalities: hemodialysis, peritoneal and CAPD*.

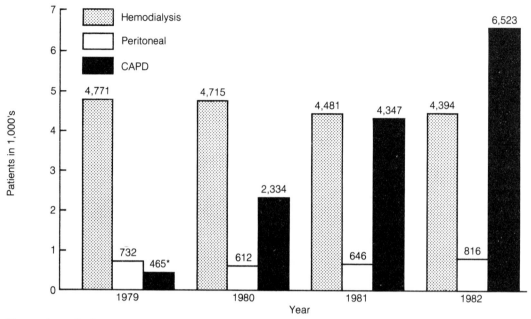

*Payment began for CAPD in 9/79. Reportings for CAPD probably misrepresented as "Peritoneal"
Source: *ESRD Medical Information System 1979, 1980, 1981 and 1982 Facility Surveys;* secondary source: *Annual Medicare Report,* 1982

TABLE 5–9.   Annual Distribution of Self-care Dialysis Patients

TREATMENT SETTING	1979	1980	1981	1982
Home	5,968	7,661	9,474	11,733
In-center	620	781	1,038	1,071
Training	519	521	495	588
Total:	7,107	8,963	11,007	13,392
Total dialysis population (%)	15 7	17 1	18 7	20 4

Source: *Annual Medicare Report,* 1982

COSTS

The type and amount of service payment and the amount for ESRD services in 1982 are shown in Table 5–12. The table shows reimbursement made by the Medicare program for services provided to ESRD patients in 1982. Although the outpatient expenditure was higher than inpatient, outpatient service is cheaper than inpatient. The larger number for outpatient services reflects the fact that many more patients receive outpatient than inpatient care.

TABLE 5–10. Mortality Rates (per 1,000 ESRD Dialysis Patients per Year) for the Dialysis Study Population Whose Date of First Reported Dialysis Was 9/73 or Later, Followed to Death, Transplant, or 9/81, by Age, Race, and Sex, and Adjusted for These Factors*

AGE (Years)	WHITE MALE (56453)[†]	WHITE FEMALE (46050)	NON WHITE MALE (25620)	NON WHITE FEMALE (24088)	TOTAL (152211)
<20	63.3	64.1	64.4	81.6	65.6
20–24	75.4	90.4	76.7	87.6	81.6
25–29	104.9	105.7	85.4	98.3	100.2
30–34	132.4	120.4	99.1	99.1	117.5
35–39	146.8	130.3	110.8	102.7	127.8
40–44	156.6	126.8	119.1	110.4	132.0
45–49	170.8	142.5	147.0	123.9	149.3
50–54	182.0	151.3	167.0	153.4	164.4
55–59	212.0	180.6	190.5	176.8	192.3
60–64	247.7	210.7	231.8	196.7	225.4
65–69	310.2	275.3	274.8	263.9	287.7
70–74	381.3	309.2	323.1	302.9	340.4
75+	490.8	444.3	443.9	347.5	454.2
Total	228.3	193.9	178.5	174.3	
Age-adjusted	142.1	128.9	126.7	125.2	
Age, race, and sex adjusted					130.4

*Adjusted to the total U.S. population in 1970
†Total number of person-years included
Source: *Annual Medicare Report*, 1982

The cost of services varies geographically. When it is higher than the ESRD reimbursement, providers can file for greater reimbursement as an exception to the normal rate level. The states that contributed the greatest proportion of exception requests were New York, Pennsylvania, Illinois, Michigan, Wisconsin, and California (Fig. 5–10).

KIDNEY TRANSPLANTS

The data on dialysis mortality underscore the need for a kidney in many renal failure patients. Kidneys for transplant are obtained from cadavers and from living, related donors. Because HLA antigens are exactly the same in 25% of all siblings, kidneys donated by a sibling are the most successful followed by those from other relatives. Kidneys from unrelated cadavers, matched for histocompatibility are least successful, e.g., subject to more intense rejection.

Before a kidney is removed from a living, related donor, he or she is evaluated for disease and for normal renal function since nephrectomy will deprive the donor of excess renal capacity. Kidneys obtained from cadavers are usually obtained from brain-dead

TABLE 5–11. Modified Life Table Analyses for the Dialysis Study Population Whose First Dialysis Was 9/73 or After (follow-up is to death, transplant, or 9/81)

	INTERVAL (YEAR)*	LX†	DEATHS	SURVIVAL‡	SURVIVAL**
Total	0	78786	13995	0.80 (0.81)	0.80 (0.81)
	1	48578	7739	0.82 (0.83)	0.66 (0.68)
	2	29853	4316	0.84 (0.85)	0.55 (0.57)
	3	18160	2352	0.85 (0.86)	0.47 (0.49)
	4	10886	1265	0.86 (0.87)	0.40 (0.43)
	5	5922	607	0.87 (0.88)	0.35 (0.38)
	6	2860	265	0.87 (0.88)	0.30 (0.33)
	7	907	54	0.89 (0.90)	0.27 (0.30)
White males	0	31010	6016	0.78 (0.80)	0.78 (0.80)
	1	18308	3277	0.80 (0.81)	0.62 (0.65)
	2	10908	1821	0.81 (0.82)	0.51 (0.53)
	3	6459	945	0.83 (0.85)	0.42 (0.45)
	4	3779	486	0.85 (0.86)	0.36 (0.39)
	5	2013	228	0.86 (0.87)	0.30 (0.34)
	6	953	99	0.85 (0.87)	0.26 (0.29)
	7	313	17	0.90 (0.91)	0.23 (0.26
White females	0	23656	4187	0.80 (0.81)	0.80 (0.81)
	1	14523	2219	0.82 (0.84)	0.66 (0.68)
	2	9089	1234	0.85 (0.85)	0.56 (0.58)
	3	5597	671	0.86 (0.87)	0.48 (0.50)
	4	3370	354	0.87 (0.88)	0.42 (0.44)
	5	1847	173	0.88 (0.89)	0.37 (0.39)
	6	888	73	0.88 (0.89)	0.33 (0.35)
	7	289	20	0.87 (0.88)	0.29 (0.38)
Nonwhite males	0	12655	1979	0.83 (0.84)	0.83 (0.84)
	1	8124	1175	0.84 (0.85)	0.69 (0.72)
	2	5054	643	0.85 (0.87)	0.59 (0.62)
	3	3135	400	0.85 (0.87)	0.50 (0.54)
	4	1908	223	0.86 (0.87)	0.43 (0.47)
	5	1031	103	0.87 (0.89)	0.38 (0.42)
	6	500	38	0.89 (0.90)	0.34 (0.38)
	7	172	13	0.86 (0.87)	0.29 (0.33)
Nonwhite females	0	11465	1813	0.83 (0.84)	0.83 (0.84)
	1	7623	1068	0.84 (0.85)	0.70 (0.71)
	2	4002	618	0.85 (0.86)	0.59 (0.62)
	3	2969	336	0.87 (0.88)	0.52 (0.54)
	4	1829	202	0.87 (0.88)	0.45 (0.47)
	5	1031	103	0.88 (0.88)	0.39 (0.42)
	6	519	55	0.84 (0.85)	0.33 (0.36)
	7	133	4	0.94 (0.95)	0.31 (0.34)

*Interval from date of entry into analysis
†Number of patients alive at the start of the specified interval
‡Crude and relative survival rates for each interval; relative survival rates given in parentheses
**Cumulative crude and relative survival rates by interval from date of entry; relative survival rates given in parentheses
Source: *NIH, National Cancer Institute;* secondary source: *Annual Medicare Report,* 1982

FIG. 5–9.   Major reasons for changes in the number of patients treated by Medicare certified suppliers of ESRD services, 1979–1982

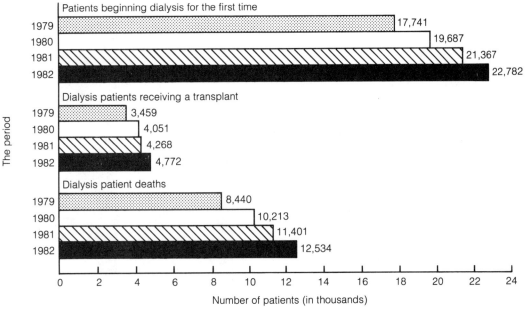

Source: *ESRD Medical Information System 1979, 1980, 1981 and 1982 Facility Surveys;* secondary source: *Annual Medicare Report,* 1982

TABLE 5–12.   End-stage Renal Disease Program Highlights December 31, 1982: Reimbursement

TYPE OF PAYMENT	AMOUNT OF PAYMENT (MILLIONS)*
Inpatient	$ 505.2
Outpatient	777.3
Physician/supplier	348.5
Home health/skilled nursing facility	6.4
Total	$1637.4

*Not final figures
Source: *Annual Medicare Report,* 1982

persons who were otherwise healthy before death. Cadaveric kidneys are preserved by special cooling solutions but must nevertheless be transplanted within 24 hours of their removal. Another, more complex preservative technique permits transplant within 72 hours.

Before transplant surgery, recipients are often treated with antibiotics to prevent infection. They are always treated with immu-

FIG. 5–10. Comparison by state of exception requests—1982

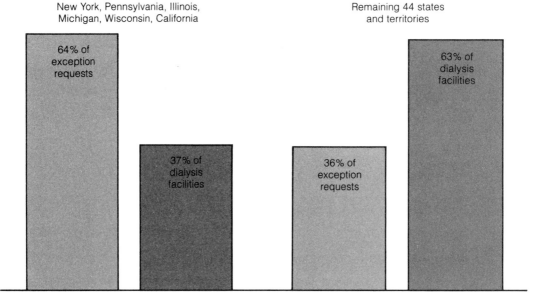

Source: *Bureau of Eligibility, Reimbursement and Coverage Program Data HCFA;* secondary source: *Annual Medicare Report,* 1982

nosuppressants, such as azathioprine, cyclophosphamide, prednisone, and more recently cyclosporin A. The last-named drug has shown great promise as an effective and specific immunosuppressant. Specific immunosuppression is critical to the survival of transplant patients because broad immunosuppression not specific to just the transplant organ antigens leads to infection, hepatitis, and even cancer in recipients.

Yet, without immunosuppression—even broad suppression in many cases—the transplanted organ will be rejected, often within 3 to 4 months after transplantation. If the prime rejection period is passed successfully and no rejection crisis ensues, renal patients can be maintained on low doses of immunosuppressant drugs that do not have adverse effects.

Changes in the number of patients awaiting a kidney transplant vs. the number who received one for the years 1979–1982 are shown in Figure 5–11. Whereas a large proportion of waiting patients received transplants in 1979 and 1980, the gap widened by 1982 when only 79.7% received a kidney compared to 87.4% for 1979 and 92.6% in 1980.

The number and proportion of kidney transplants by donor type, either living or cadaver, for each ESRD region is shown in Figure 5–12.

FIG. 5–11. Patients awaiting transplants vs. transplants performed

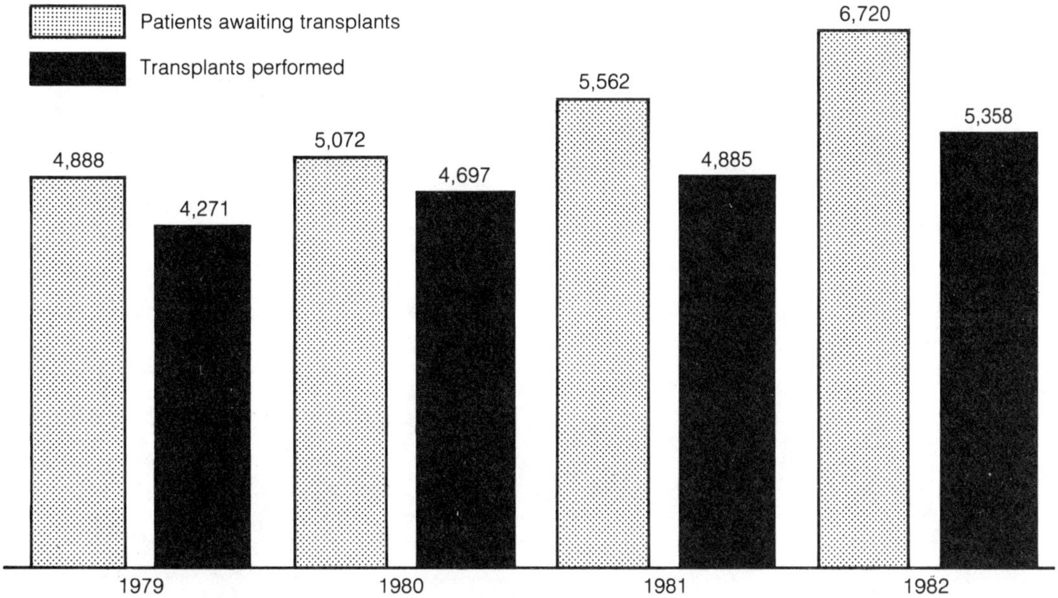

Source: *ESRD Medical Information System 1979, 1980, 1981 and 1982 Facility Surveys*; secondary source: *Annual Medicare Report, 1982*

The patients receiving a kidney transplant were highest in the states of California and New York (Table 5–13). Note that most kidneys were from cadavers.

Preventing rejection of a transplanted kidney is a major therapeutic concern. Since the introduction of cyclosporin, graft retention rates have improved. As of 1979, the retention rate is much higher for those who receive a kidney from a related donor at 69% after 3 years vs. 45% for those with a kidney from an unrelated donor (Table 5–14). As can be seen in Table 5–15, the 1- and 3-year retention rates are higher in general for females than males, better for whites than blacks and higher for those between age 21 and 30 years than those either older and (in most cases) younger.

MORTALITY

The mortality rates for transplant patients according to age, sex, and race measured at death, transplant failure plus 3 months, and termination of entitlement or until 1981 are presented in Table 5–16. The mortality rate per 1,000 patients both before and after age adjustment was highest for nonwhite females in many age

FIG. 5–12. Transplant types by network—1982

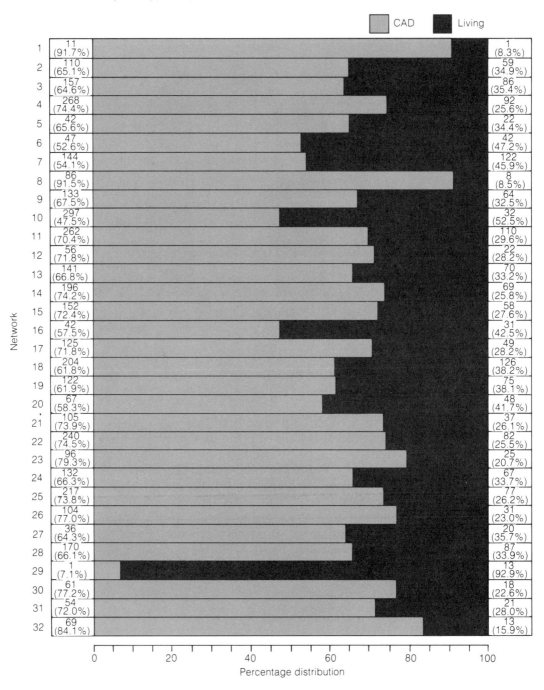

Source: *ESRD Medical Information System 1982 Facility Surveys*

TABLE 5–13. Transplants Performed During 1982, by State

STATE	FACILITIES SURVEYED REPORTING	TOTAL PATIENTS	TOTAL TRANSPLANTS	LIVING DONOR	CADAVERIC DONOR
Alabama	1	132	132	54	78
Arizona	4	62	62	30	32
Arkansas	2	17	17	15	2
California	13	602	603	178	425
Colorado	1	44	44	11	33
Connecticut	2	56	56	20	36
Washington, D.C.	5	121	121	25	96
Florida	4	197	197	75	122
Georgia	4	75	75	31	44
Hawaii	1	12	12	1	11
Illinois	7	210	210	58	152
Indiana	2	73	73	31	42
Iowa	1	59	60	7	53
Kansas	2	58	58	14	44
Kentucky	2	79	79	19	60
Louisiana	5	78	78	22	56
Maine	1	22	22	3	19
Maryland	3	75	75	21	54
Massachusetts	7	221	221	81	140
Michigan	10	267	267	69	198
Minnesota	3	266	266	122	144
Mississippi	1	30	30	1	29
Missouri	6	139	139	50	89
Nebraska	1	34	34	1	33
New Jersey	3	82	82	13	69
New Mexico	1	27	27	12	15
New York	13	426	429	108	321
North Carolina	5	138	142	37	105
Ohio	9	294	298	111	187
Oklahoma	4	44	44	17	27
Oregon	1	76	76	22	54
Pennsylvania	8	317	318	68	250
Puerto Rico	1	14	14	13	1
South Carolina	1	40	40	17	23
Tennessee	2	168	168	71	97
Texas	8	372	372	110	262
Utah	1	20	20	11	9
Vermont	1	14	14	3	11
Virginia	4	79	79	18	61
Washington	4	92	93	37	56
Wisconsin	2	211	211	70	141
Total	156	5,343	5,358	1,677	3,681

Source: *ESRD Medical Information System 1982 Facility Surveys*

TABLE 5–14.   Graft Retention Rates by Year of Transplantation

CATEGORY	UNRELATED DONOR TRANSPLANTS			RELATED DONOR TRANSPLANTS		
Percent retained to:	1 year	3 years	Cases entered	1 year	3 years	Cases entered
1977	52 ± 1%	40 ± 1%	1202	70 ± 2%	61 ± 2%	857
1978	53 ± 1	41 ± 1	1845	73 ± 1	63 ± 2	940
1979	56 ± 1	45 ± 1	2149	76 ± 1	69 ± 2	895
1980	61 ± 1	–	2395	82 ± 1	–	797

NOTE: The uncertainties are standard errors.
Source: *NIH, National Institute of Allergy and Infectious Diseases;* secondary source: *Annual Medicare Report,* 1982

TABLE 5–15.   Graft Retention Rates for the Various Demographic Categories

CATEGORY	UNRELATED DONOR TRANSPLANTS			RELATED DONOR TRANSPLANTS		
Percent retained to:	1 year	3 years	Cases entered	1 year	3 years	Cases entered
Overall	56 + 1%	45 + 1%	7591	75 + 1%	67 + 1%	3489
Male	55 + 1	44 + 1	4808	74 + 1	65 + 1	2076
Female	58 + 1	46 + 1	2776	78 + 1	71 + 1	1409
			7584			3485
Black	50 ± 1	37 ± 1	1624	64 ± 3	55 ± 3	364
White	58 ± 1	47 ± 1	5578	79 ± 1	69 ± 1	2901
			7202			3265
Age = 0–10 yrs	58 ± 4	46 ± 4	155	80 ± 3	71 ± 4	149
11–20	59 ± 2	46 ± 2	843	77 ± 2	68 ± 2	662
21–30	59 ± 1	48 ± 1	1790	79 ± 1	72 ± 1	1179
31–40	56 ± 1	44 ± 1	2010	74 ± 2	66 ± 2	797
41–50	54 ± 1	42 ± 1	1737	69 ± 2	58 ± 2	490
Over 50	52 ± 1	41 ± 1	1049	68 ± 3	60 ± 3	207
			7584			3484

*The discrepancies in the totals are the result of exclusion of cases with missing data. In addition, results for the small, heterogeneous group of persons other than black or white are not shown.
Note: The uncertainties are standard errors.
Source: *NIH, National Institute of Allergy and Infectious Diseases*

brackets followed by non-white and white males. The high non-white female rate was skewed, perhaps by the very high rate for these women between age 65 and 69 years, which was based on only five cases. Generally, the mortality rate for each sex/race group was lower at younger age levels although exceptions can be found among nonwhite males ages 40 to 49 years and for nonwhite females between age 30 and 34 years.

Life table analysis indicates that survival chances improve once a patient has survived the first year after transplant. They rise from 85% to 89% during the first year to 93% and 97% by the third posttransplant year (Table 5–17).

TABLE 5–16. Mortality Rates (per 1,000 ESRD transplant patients, per year) for the Renal Transplantation Population Whose Date of First Reported Transplant was 7/73 or Later, Followed to Death, Date of Transplant Failure Plus 3 Months, Termination of Entitlement, or 9/81, by Age, Race, and Sex, and Adjusted* for These Factors

AGE	WHITE MALE (11076)[†]	WHITE FEMALE (7532)	NONWHITE MALE (2864)	NONWHITE FEMALE (1480)	TOTAL (22952)
Less than 20	54.2	45.8	52.3	106.8	53.2
20–24	54.7	43.1	79.5	40.1	52.2
25–29	53.1	63.6	74.7	95.5	61.8
30–34	71.5	79.1	71.5	154.4	79.4
35–39	106.3	108.2	124.8	110.6	110.0
40–44	107.9	108.0	151.3	149.3	118.8
45–49	177.5	138.1	218.6	178.6	172.5
50–54	178.9	169.1	162.8	203.9	175.7
55–59	198.3	155.3	241.4	197.0	188.8
60–64	223.2	90.9	243.9		197.5
65–69	257.1	94.3[‡]		678.0[‡]	173.6
70–74	129.9[‡]	202.0[‡]	83.3[‡]		141.5[†]
75+	800.0[‡]	–0–[‡]			224.7[†]
Total	99.6	86.4	123.2	131.8	
Age-adjusted	126.6	79.4	99.3	147.4	
Age, race, and sex adjusted					113.2

*Adjusted to the total U.S. population in 1970
[†]Total number of person-years included
[‡]Rate based upon 5 or fewer deaths
Source: *Annual Medicare Report,* 1982

TABLE 5–17. Modified Life Table Analyses for the Renal Transplantation Population Whose First Transplant was 7/73 or After (follow-up is to death, date of transplant failure plus 3 months, termination of entitlement, or 9/81, whichever occurred first)

POPULATION	INTERVAL (YEAR)*	LX[†]	DEATHS	SURVIVAL[‡]	SURVIVAL**
Total	0	18590	1968	0.88 (0.88)	0.88 (0.88)
	1	11943	218	0.97 (0.97)	0.86 (0.86)
	2	3888	116	9.96 (0.96)	0.82 (0.82)
White males	0	8897	935	0.88 (0.88)	0.88 (0.88)
	1	5737	115	0.97 (0.97)	0.85 (0.86)
	2	1902	53	0.96 (0.97)	0.82 (0.83)
White females	0	5884	567	0.89 (0.89)	0.89 (0.89)
	1	3995	53	0.98 (0.98)	0.87 (0.88)
	2	1317	31	0.97 (0.97)	0.85 (0.85)
Non-white males	0	2515	296	0.86 (0.89)	0.86 (0.87)
	1	1432	32	0.97 (0.97)	0.83 (0.84)
	2	445	25	0.93 (0.93)	0.77 (0.78)
Non-white females	0	1294	170	0.85 (0.85)	0.85 (0.85)
	1	779	18	0.96 (0.97)	0.82 (0.82)
	2	224	7	0.96 (0.96)	0.78 (0.79)

*Interval from date of entry into analysis
[†]Number of patients alive at start of specified interval
[‡]Crude and relative survival rates for each interval; relative survival rates given in parentheses
**Cumulative crude and relative survival rates by interval from date of entry; relative survival rates given in parentheses
Source: *NIH, National Cancer Institute*

COSTS

The cost of obtaining a kidney for transplant from the several independent suppliers who serve major cities is summarized in Table 5–18. The cost reported by different agencies varies considerably, even within one region.

The acquisition cost of cadaveric kidneys paid by hospitals (Table 5–19) is typically $500 and $3,000 less than the charge to recipients (Table 5–20)

TABLE 5–18.   1982 Kidney Acquisition Costs Reported by Independent Organ Procurement Agencies by Region

REGION	COST/KIDNEY
Boston	$ 9,831
New York	1,331*
	6,055
	7,388
Philadelphia	1,787
	6,222
	7,886
Atlanta	0†
	4,040
	5,184
	5,672
	12,157
	13,861
	14,064
Chicago	5,947
	7,078
	8,170†
	8,432
	11,075
Dallas	6,043
	7,216
	7,895
	8,737
Kansas City	6,019
	8,209
	9,236
Denver	0‡
San Francisco	1,923†
	9,211
Seattle	7,483

*Limited service OPAS
†First year of activity
‡No activity
Source: *Medicare Fiscal Intermediaries' Reimbursement Files*

TABLE 5–19.   Kidney Acquisition Costs: Average and Range of Estimated Costs for Cadaveric Donor Kidneys for 1982 by Region

REGION	HIGH	LOW	AVERAGE
Boston	$ 8,900	$1,346	$ 5,350
New York	14,631	1,977	6,904
Philadelphia	18,612	4,851	7,547
Atlanta	10,780	3,143	7,304
Chicago	27,300	2,388	8,247
Dallas	8,235	3,919	5,863
Kansas City	22,360	5,766	13,287
Denver	7,726	3,673	5,699
San Francisco	10,761	5,226	7,697
Seattle	11,787	7,575	8,464
National	14,109	3,986	7,636

Source: *Annual Medicare Report,* 1982

TABLE 5–20.   Kidney Acquisition Charges: Average and Range for Cadaveric Donor Kidneys for 1982 by Region

REGION	HIGH	LOW	AVERAGE
Boston	$10,500	$1,950	$ 6,771
New York	15,000	2,400	8,307
Philadelphia	19,800	3,975	9,357
Atlanta	11,165	3,590	7,961
Chicago	30,000	2,400	9,214
Dallas	9,800	1,500	6,659
Kansas City	24,000	7,000	14,698
Denver	8,547	4,100	6,324
San Francisco	13,000	7,100	8,905
Seattle	14,920	7,500	9,980
National	$15,673	$4,152	$ 8,818

Source: *Annual Medicare Report,* 1982

The acquisition cost of a donor kidney from a living relative is considerably higher than that from a cadaver (Table 5–21). The difference between the acquisition cost of a related donor kidney and the charge to the patient is between $300 and $3,000 as comparison of Tables 5–21 and 5–22 indicates.

HOSPITAL STAYS

The hospital stays for ESRD patients, transplant and nontransplant, totaled 97,023 (Table 5–23). The average charge per stay was $4,904. The total charge amounted to $475,801,000, with reimbursement for covered days equalling $341,536,000. Although hos-

TABLE 5–21. Kidney Acquisition Costs: Average and Range of Estimated Costs for Living Related Donor Kidneys for 1982 by Region

REGION	HIGH	LOW	AVERAGE
Boston	$ 9,831	$1,780	$ 5,065
New York	14,631	1,977	6,978
Philadelphia	18,612	4,851	8,202
Atlanta	18,086	3,940	7,649
Chicago	30,030	2,931	8,356
Dallas	11,642	3,563	6,101
Kansas City	22,360	5,766	12,010
Denver	8,990	6,271	7,630
San Francisco	11,803	2,678	7,922
Seattle	11,787	4,137	7,777
National	$15,777	$3,789	$ 7,769

Source: *Medicare Fiscal Intermediaries' Reimbursement Files*

TABLE 5–22. Kidney Acquisition Charges: Average and Range for Living Related Donor Kidneys for 1982 by Region

REGION	HIGH	LOW	AVERAGE
Boston	$11,300	$2,000	$ 6,464
New York	15,000	2,400	8,398
Philadelphia	19,800	5,600	10,301
Atlanta	20,240	4,500	8,434
Chicago	33,000	3,300	9,128
Dallas	14,000	3,000	7,050
Kansas City	23,075	7,000	13,225
Denver	9,946	7,000	8,473
San Francisco	13,550	3,500	9,132
Seattle	14,920	4,500	9,480
National	$17,483	$4,260	$ 9,009

Source: *Annual Medicare Report, 1982*

pital stays related to transplant procedures accounted for only 4% of all stays of ESRD patients studied, the transplant stay charges comprised 21% of their total hospital charge.

The hospitalization rate, measured as the number of discharges for ESRD patients, was estimated according to sex, race, and age during 1980 and 1981 when transplant patients were excluded. The rate was highest for those age 65 years and older, females, and non-whites (Table 5–24). Average length of stay was longest for the elderly. Note too that the elderly patients, while fewer at only 15,020 compared to 21,951 middle-aged patients, accounted for more discharges in 1981. Therefore, many elderly have had more than one hospital discharge within the years studied.

TABLE 5–23. Charges, Estimated Reimbursements and Average Length of Stay for Transplants and Nontransplant Hospital Stays: 1980

	ALL STAYS	TRANSPLANTS STAYS	NONTRANSPLANTS STAYS		
			All	Nonsurgical	Surgical
Stays (%)*	97,023	4,227	92,796	57,548	35, 248
	100%	4%	96%	59%	36%
Charges	$475,801	$102,243	$373,558	$148,041	$225,517
(in 1,000s)(%)	100%	21%	79%	31%	47%
Charges/stay	$4,904	$24,188	$4,026	$2,572	$6,398
Estimated					
reimbursement	$341,536	$81,513	$260,023	$103,064	$156,959
(1,000s)(%)	100%	24%	76%	30%	46%
Estimated					
reimbursement/stay	$3,520	$19,284	$2,802	$1,791	$4,453
Covered days (%)	1,120,489	127,655	992,834	566,060	426,774
	100%	11%	89%	51%	38%
Average length of					
stay (covered days)	11.5	30.2	10.7	9.8	12.1

*Percentages may not add up to 100 due to rounding.
Source: *1980 Medpar 20 Percent Sample of Hospital Stays*

Hospital stay data for ESRD patients, including transplant patients for 1980 and 1981, are presented in Table 5–25. Again, those older than age 65 years were fewer than middle-aged patients but accounted for more discharges and more days of care than any other age group except those younger than age 24 years who also had the longest average stay.

Survival of renal patients 3 years after initiating end-stage treatment was greatest for those who received a related donor kidney transplant (Table 5–26). Those who received an unrelated kidney showed the next best survival, whereas those on dialysis came in a poor third with a rate of only 54% to 57% 3 years after beginning treatment.

The best survival rates among the various age, sex, and racial groups who received either dialysis or transplant was reported for those between ages 11 and 30 years who had received a related-donor transplant. Except for people in certain age intervals transplant patients showed better survival in all demographic categories than did dialysis patients. Black transplant patients fared less well than white, but black dialysis patients did better than white dialysis patients (Table 5–27).

The great expense and debility caused by ESRD prompt efforts at prevention. Many renal disorders leading to failure such as the ones that are immuno-mediated are not well understood by current science. As yet, they are not preventable. But renal failure that follows streptoccocal or renal infections and episodes that follow the inges-

TABLE 5–24. Hospitalization Rates for Medicare ESRD Beneficiaries by Age, Sex, and Race; 1980 and 1981 (excluding transplant patients)

PATIENTS	1980				1981			
	ESRD Persons (July 1)	Discharges 1,000	Days of Care/1,000	Average Stay	ESRD Persons (July 1)	Discharges/ 1,000	Days of Care/1,000	Average Stay
Total	53,896	1,591	17,320	10.9	59,986	1,570	16,718	10.7
Age:								
0–24	3,315	1,137	11,529	10.1	3,650	1,332	12,848	9.6
25–44	13,610	1,393	14,534	10.4	15,641	1,405	13,947	9.9
45–64	21,951	1,608	17,074	10.6	24,595	1,606	16,677	10.4
65+	15,020	1,845	21,480	11.6	16,100	1,727	20,351	11.8
Sex:								
Male	29,352	1,503	16,203	10.8	32,620	1,487	15,490	10.4
Female	24,544	1,696	18,655	11.0	27,366	1,668	18,183	10.9
Race:								
White	36,462	1,593	17,384	10.9	40,151	1,583	16,895	10.7
Black	14,350	1,630	17,775	10.9	16,222	1,588	17,081	10.7
Other/Unknown	3,088	1,376	14,424	10.5	3,617	1,335	13,395	10.0

Source: ESRD Medical Information System Inpatient Stay Records, 1980 and 1981

TABLE 5–25. Hospitalization Rates for Medicare ESRD Beneficiaries by Age, Sex, and Race; 1980 and 1981 (including transplant patients)

PATIENTS	1980				1981			
	ESRD Persons (July 1)	Discharges/ 1,000	Days of Care/1,000	Average Stay	ESRD Persons (July 1)	Discharges/ 1,000	Days of Care/1,000	Average Stay
Total	57,814	1,678	19,381	11.5	64,059	1,653	18,691	11.3
Age:								
0–24	4,277	1,604	19,559	12.2	4,650	1,737	20,243	11.7
25–44	15,621	1,570	18,668	11.9	17,732	1,566	17,802	11.4
45–64	22,888	1,656	18,444	11.1	25,568	1,651	17,967	10.9
65+	15,028	1,846	21,498	11.6	16,109	1,728	20,368	11.8
Sex:								
Male	31,804	1,608	18,628	11.6	35,168	1,587	17,822	11.2
Female	26,010	1,763	20,301	11.5	28,891	1,733	19,747	11.4
Race:								
White	39,459	1,695	19,689	11.6	43,266	1,681	19,116	11.4
Black	15,028	1,679	19,194	11.4	16,927	1,634	18,360	11.2
Other/Unknown	3,331	1,470	16,550	11.3	3,870	1,422	15,363	10.8

Source: ESRD Medical Information System Inpatient Stay Records, 1980 and 1981

TABLE 5–26. Patient Survival Rates by Year of Onset of Treatment

| CATEGORY: | DIALYSIS | | | TRANSPLANTATION | | | | | |
| | | | | Unrelated Donor Transplants | | | Related Donor Transplants | | |
Percent surviving to:	1 year	3 years	Cases entered	1 year	3 years	Cases entered	1 year	3 years	Cases entered
1977	82 ± .3%	57 ± .5%	16,501	87 ± 1%	79 ± 1%	1203	94 ± 1%	89 ± 1%	857
1978	82 ± .5	54 ± .5	14,301	84 ± 1	75 ± 1	1849	94 ± 1	89 ± 1	944
1979	81 ± .3	55 ± .5	16,605	85 ± 1	77 ± 1	2151	95 ± 1	92 ± 1	895
1980	81 ± .3	—	17,863	87 ± 1	—	2399	95 ± 1	—	797

Note: The uncertainties are standard errors.
Source: NIH, National Institute of Allergy and Infectious Diseases

TABLE 5–27.   Patient Survival Rates for the Various Demographic Categories

| | DIALYSIS | | | TRANSPLANTATION | | | | | |
| | | | | UNRELATED DONOR TRANSPLANTS | | | RELATED DONOR TRANSPLANTS | | |
CATEGORY Percent surviving to:	1 year	3 years	Cases entered	1 year	3 years	Cases entered	1 year	3 years	Cases entered
Overall	81 ± .2%	56 ± .3%	65,270	86 ± .4%	78 ± .5%	7595	95 ± .4%	91 ± .6%	3491
Male	81 ± .3	55 ± .4	36,600	86 ± .6	77 ± 1	4818	95 ± .5	90 ± 1	2079
Female	82 ± .4	58 ± .4	28,581	86 ± 1	78 ± 1	2777	94 ± .6	91 ± 1	1410
			65,181			7595			3489
Black	85 ± .3	62 ± .5	17,194	86 ± 1	78 ± 1	1625	93 ± 1	87 ± 2	364
White	80 ± .2	54 ± .3	43,990	86 ± .5	77 ± 1	5588	95 ± .4	91 ± 1	2905
			61,184			7213			3269
Age = 0–10 yrs	90 ± 2	82 ± 3	601	89 ± 3	80 ± 3	155	93 ± 2	89 ± 3	150
11–20	95 ± .5	88 ± 2	2,620	92 ± 1	87 ± 1	844	97 ± 1	95 ± 1	662
21–30	91 ± .5	78 ± 1	6,240	92 ± 1	87 ± 1	1792	97 ± 1	95 ± 1	1180
31–40	89 ± .5	71 ± 1	7,883	85 ± 1	78 ± 1	2016	93 ± 1	89 ± 1	798
41–50	88 ± .4	68 ± .7	9,995	81 ± 1	70 ± 1	1737	91 ± 1	82 ± 2	490
Over 50	77 ± .2	48 ± .3	35,911	79 ± 1	68 ± 2	1051	88 ± 2	81 ± 3	208
			63,250			7595			3488

*The discrepancies in the totals are the result of exclusion of cases with missing data; in addition, results for the small, heterogeneous group of persons other than black or white are not shown.

Note: The uncertainties are standard errors.

Source: NIH, National Institute of Allergy and Infectious Diseases; secondary source: Annual Medicare Report, 1982

tion of nephrotoxic substances, such as the heavy metals and various legal and illegal drugs, can be prevented. Still, the public is generally unaware of the causes and life-threatening aspects of renal disease. Health education prevention efforts are a good start as research for more effective treatment, including better modes of dialysis, better ways to secure graft retention, and even better ways to repair damaged kidneys continues.

A Note On Methodology

This volume and the others in this series are concerned with the demographics of disease, and the disease patterns of different groups of people considered on the basis of age, sex, or cultural grouping. The study of these patterns and the causes of disease in large and small populations is called *epidemiology.*

For thousands of years, people believed that sickness was a punishment for transgressions against the gods. The pattern of sinfulness followed by sickness was evident often enough, for people seldom lived perfect lives and seldom avoided all disease. When sick, they would call for a shaman, a priest-doctor who would beg the gods through prayer and incantation to restore the sick to health.

As simplistic as this approach seems to many modern peoples, the basic impetus of early peoples was epidemiologic. They had isolated a pattern of disease and sought to avoid the scourge of disease by addressing its cause, an angry god.

Gradually, exceptions to the accepted pattern of disease were noticed. Epidemics affected virtually everyone in a community, good or bad. So, too, people began to notice other patterns of illness and linked aspects of their natural surroundings, such as their drinking water and certain foods, to the development of disease.

People also noticed that those in contact with a sick person often developed the same symptoms a few days or weeks later. Thus, a belief developed that disease could be transmitted somehow from person to person, perhaps by the movement of invisible particles traveling from the body of the sick person to that of the well one. The writings of Lucretius described this theory of contagious disease. With this pattern of disease noticed, the stage was set for the development of modern epidemiology, the science that looks for the pattern of diseases and the natural causes evidenced by that pattern.

Although the stage was set, many obstacles still had to be overcome. Autopsy examinations were forbidden through most of the Middle Ages, and everyday observational tools used by the modern physician, such as the clinical thermometer and the stethoscope, were not invented until the 17th and 18th centuries, respectively. Thus, it was difficult to diagnose the cause of death in many instances. Those who hazarded a guess were often wildly simplistic or incorrect.

Even in the 20th century, influenza, pneumonia, bronchitis, and tuberculosis have routinely been mistaken for each other. Autopsies performed in the latter part of this century finally helped to clarify mortality from this cause.

THE DEATH CERTIFICATE

Despite today's much improved knowledge of the body and disease, the problems of relying on the information entered on a death certificate are notorious. Unfortunately, mortality data reported by countries around the world are based of necessity on death-certificate entries.

In many countries, death-certificate entries represent a physician's diagnosis. But in many other countries, the cause of death is reported by the deceased's relatives to a local clerk. Even in more sophisticated countries, listing the cause of death often obscures the real pathologic profile. For example, dying is always a dualistic event resulting from the interaction of a given host and the disease agent that afflicts the host. In one person, influenza may prove fatal because he is constitutionally weak, perhaps from age or other diseases. In another person, encounter with the influenza virus would be a minor event—in no way life threatening. But the record of influenza mortality translates simply into the ferocity or danger of influenza as a disease.

The decline in measles mortality throughout much of the 20th century is another example of the confluence of several factors. Until the recent development of the measles vaccine, nothing had changed in the incidence or severity of measles. But mortality in those stricken with pneumonia, a common fatal sequel of measles, was being reduced by sulfa drugs.

Similarly, much information and understanding are lost insofar as death certificates require a listing of only one cause of death, although secondary causes can be listed on the back. Conventions have been established that priority should be given to the cause that is most often fatal, communicable or acute. But such conventions vary from country to country.

This practice becomes increasingly problematic as populations experience greater longevity, since old people often suffer from several conditions by the time they die of any one cited cause. Someone with diabetes, poor renal function, and congestive heart failure (CHF) is taxed by a cold that develops into acute bronchitis. Medication places an added burden on their kidneys. Difficulty in breathing places an extra oxygen demand on their heart, while their blood sugar is difficult to control. After a few days, their kidneys fail as does their heart and they die. Did the cold kill them? Did the bronchitis? Or was the cause of death heart failure, kidney failure, or diabetes? The physician must make a choice. In England and Wales, the death rate from bronchitis is higher than in most other countries. But these UK countries are inclined to list cases like the one described as a bronchitis death whereas other countries tend to list it as a cardiovascular death.

When a death certificate was introduced in England that asked the physician to list death "as consequence of," the number of deaths ascribed to bronchitis doubled. Deaths from nephritis in Canada and the United States doubled as well, while one-third to one-half of the deaths typically attributed to diabetes were counted for some other cause.

DIFFICULTIES OF NOMENCLATURE AND CLASSIFICATION

Beyond these difficulties are ones of nomenclature and classification. To solve these problems, an International Classification of Diseases has been established, which has been revised from time to time. The current code represents the ninth such revision. But in its attempt to standardize diagnosis from country to country, the classification has posed other problems. As knowledge of diseases has increased, the classification has gradually changed from anatomic groupings to etiologic ones. Rheumatic fever is still listed anatomically as a heart disease because it affects the heart. But if it were true to the trend, it would be listed according to cause and would be regarded as an infectious disease because we now know that rheumatic fever is caused by a bacterium and is infectious. In the fourth revision, brain tumors were removed from the category of nervous system diseases and put with neoplasms, as we realized that these tumors are the results of cancerous growth. During the fourth revision of the code, a more mysterious change was the removal of criminal abortion from accidental death to complication of pregnancy.

Over the years, as diagnosis has become more specific, deaths due to ill-defined causes have also decreased and other heretofore ill-defined diseases, such as various neoplasms, show increased mortality. As populations have aged and physicians have become accustomed to diagnosing the cause of death in the old, several degenerative diseases, such as diabetes, nephritis, ulcer, and cirrhosis have left the ill-defined category.

CENSUS PROBLEMS

In addition to classification and nomenclature complexities, elementary census biases enter the picture when countries try to calculate their mortality and morbidity rate due to different diseases. These rates are usually expressed as the number of deaths or disease cases per 100,000 population. Sometimes the rates are calculated for men and women separately or for people in different age groups separately. But census numbers are known for their underestimates of population even in advanced countries like the United States. Young children and transient males who travel for their work are often missed in population counts. The 1960 United States census missed an estimated three million people, particularly blacks. Latin Americans tend to report more 5- to 9-year-old children than 0- to 4-year-olds.

Often, information on sex is missing and when asked for their age, people tend to say they are 18 or 21 when these are the ages of majority in a country and 65 when social benefits are available to 65-year-olds. Many people between age 21 and 40 years tend to lower their age when asked. On the other hand, those who do report their true age tend to round their age, especially to even numbers or to ages divisible by five. To compensate for this tendency, researchers often use age intervals when these statistics are compiled.

SURVEYS

Data on morbidity pose yet different problems in that they are usually obtained from health department reports, review of hospital records, or sample surveys of the population. In the United States, physicians are legally obligated to report a large array of diseases, particularly infectious ones, to their health departments. The latter in turn report their data to the Atlanta Centers for Disease Control. Reports come from all of the states, but data gathered independently tend to reveal an under-reporting of disease to the Centers in many instances.

Sometimes hospital records are used for gathering data but these records are often incomplete or have incorrect entries. In addition, hospitalized patients may not reflect the typical patient with a given disease because hospitalized patients are likely to be those who are more severely ill with a specific disease or those who are intractable to less extreme forms of outpatient treatments.

Sample surveys are also subject to misleading findings, depending on how the sample is chosen and how the survey questions are constructed and asked. Data from several large government surveys have been included in this volume. Elaborate statistical sampling methods have been employed to ensure that the surveys are representative. But the questions sometimes fail to elicit pertinent and interesting information. One example can be found in the discussion in *Cardiovascular Disease* that deals with cerebrovascular disease.

A sample of people were asked about their limitation of normal activity due, presumably, to illness. Some were people who had suffered a stroke; others had not. The stroke victims generally showed greater limitation of activity. But these same people were also generally older and perhaps infirm because of other health conditions. There was no indication that their limitation of activity was specifically related to their stroke event. Thus, we do not know, in light of this particular study, how much dysfunction is caused by stroke in the general population compared to other disability conditions of able-bodied people.

The operations and procedures, together with hospital utilization and physician office visits for people with various diagnoses discussed in this work, were obtained from large government studies, such as the National Ambulatory Care Survey and the National Hospital Discharge Survey, which are conducted annually or periodically. Again the focus of these surveys is not always constant from one to another. Comparison of data from an early survey, such as the NHANES I Nutrition Survey with data on some variables measured by a later survey, such as the NHANES II Survey, is not always possible.

RANDOM VARIABILITY

The perspicacious reader must also realize that health data gathered through survey studies are always subject to a certain amount of random variability. More than a century ago, scientists found to their chagrin that whenever any entity is measured multiple times, the measurement varies. This is true even when the measurement is taken by the same person each time using the same instrument in the same way.

In astronomy, this variability came to be known as the personal equation. But this same kind of variability occurs when one obtains data from a random sample presumably representative of a population of interest. Another random sample surveyed in the same way and equally representative typically yields slightly different results. This variability is called the standard error of a particular study.

The importance of keeping in mind that every sample surveyed has a standard error comes into play when comparisons of data expressed as averages are made. Luckily, the standard error of studies is often small; hence, fairly large differences among groups can be accepted as true differences in reality and not merely the reflection of sampling variability.

When reported differences are small, however, one should not conclude that there is in fact a real difference between two groups unless one knows that the standard error of the study samples is smaller than the small reported difference. For a more detailed explanation of sampling variability, see my article, "Randomization and optimal design," *Journal of Chronic Diseases* 36:606–609, 1983.

CRUDE AND AGE-ADJUSTED DATA

Another factor that good health surveys take into account is the age of the groups compared. Clearly, if the blacks interviewed in a study sample were on average 10 years younger than white subjects, one would be mistaken to conclude that whites smoke more than blacks. Obviously, members of groups that smoke to the same degree will show one smoking longer than the other if the members of one group are older than those of the other. The way to correct for age differences when age is likely to affect whether one has an illness or has followed a particular pattern for some time is to compare age-adjusted samples. You will note throughout this volume that crude rates are given as are age-adjusted rates when they are relevant and available.

Since the rates of mortality and morbidity vary among people of different ages, sex, races, and sometimes ethnic and religious backgrounds—particularly in the United States—one has to be mindful of differences in these groups that may account for their differing disease rates. Age is clearly one of these differences that needs to be adjusted for when comparing data. The average and median ages of the black United States population are considerably lower than the white population. Thus, we would expect to see a lower rate of old-age degenerative disease among blacks than among whites when there is no age adjustment. When age is adjusted for or the rate at the same age is compared, epidemiologists have discovered that blacks actually have a higher rate of hypertension than whites.

Another factor not as easily corrected for is access to and utilization of medical resources. If a particular group, such as blacks, are economically less able or socially less inclined to seek medical care when sick, they may ultimately reflect a higher mortality rate from their diseases or a greater morbidity rate as their untreated conditions grow more severe. The higher mortality in such situations should not be regarded as an indication that the higher mortality group has the disease to a greater extent. In other words, blacks may not have more cancer than whites, but they may have a higher cancer mortality rate because they do not receive an early diagnosis or follow treatment regimens for economic or social reasons.

Some researchers speculate that males have a higher general mortality rate than females in part because they tend to seek less medical help for their ailments and fail to follow prescribed treatment regimens for psychological reasons or because it is not convenient for them to see a physician due to career demands.

Aside from the differences in the groups just discussed, differences also exist in groups that may explain why disease does indeed occur more often in some groups than in others. In fact, this is the basic logic of epidemiology and the real incentive for keeping track of vital statistics. Epidemiologists seek to isolate patterns in disease to determine possible pathologic causes.

TELLING PATTERNS

Once it is determined that members of one group are sick and those of another are not, epidemiologists study factors that may be affecting the groups differently. One of the earliest of these investigations was conducted by the physician John Snow, who investigated cholera in London between 1848 and 1854. At that time, different parts of London were supplied with water by different companies. Snow noticed that the cholera cases were confined to areas supplied by two specific water companies. In contrast to the others these two obtained their water from a very polluted section of the Thames River.

One of the companies changed its source farther upriver and when water pipes were laid in the city, its pipes were alternated with those of the other Thames River company such that each supplied every other house in an area of London that they both served. Snow counted the number of houses in the district served by each company and the number of cholera cases that developed in houses served by each company.

The resulting rates were greatly different, with a much higher rate of cholera in the houses served by the company that was still drawing its water from the polluted source.

This classic study reflects a design referred to as the case control method. This form of research is especially important and useful when one is trying to determine the possible cause of a disease. It has been employed widely and added to our medical knowledge in ways such as the discovery that infant deformities were in the offspring of women who had nothing in common other than ingestion of thalidomide during their pregnancy to the studies that showed a much higher incidence of lung cancer among smokers than among nonsmokers.

Much of the work that has revealed the risk factors for various cancers were obtained from case control studies that compared people with cancer to a group of people without cancer, the control group, which was matched in age, sex, and so on with the disease or case group. Middle-aged women in Aurora, Illinois, were reported to have bone cancer more than women in surrounding communities. They seemed like the other women except that they had all worked at a radium dial watch factory in Aurora some years previously, whereas none of the cancer-free control group had worked with the radium. The conclusion was that exposure to radioactive material is a risk factor for developing bone cancer.

Because of modern developments in statistical analysis, researchers also determine possible risk factors when more than one is operative. Such analysis would be used with large cross-sectional community studies that record the prevalence of a disease and other characteristics of the population. The Framingham heart study was of this sort. It revealed that people with heart disease tend to have hypertension, elevated cholesterol readings, and a history of smoking more than those who do not suffer from heart disease.

A follow-up study conducted for several years is currently recording the practices of the offspring of the original study population and the development of heart disease among them. This type of study is called a cohort incidence study because it looks for the development of disease over time. Expensive and lengthy, it is also sometimes impractical.

Each of these designs is useful when one is trying to find the cause of a disease, especially a disease that develops slowly over time. Another type of design that is useful to determine the best form of treatment for a disease is the clinical trial. Some professionals erroneously regard this design as more scientific than the others because the investigator has some control over the exposure of the test sample to a given factor, a treatment of some sort, but this view is incorrect. The randomized controlled trial is subject to many of the same biases as the other designs that I discuss in my article, "The case control or retrospective study in Retrospect," *Journal of Clinical Pharmacology* 21:269–274, July 1981. The debate is moot, however, because the clinical trial cannot be used to determine the cause of a disease. No one can ethically subject healthy people to a factor suspected of causing a disease.

An early example of a clinical trial that *did* test various treatments and also determined the cause of a disease was an investigation made by James Lind into the treatment of scurvy among English sailors in 1747. Sailors long away at sea were afflicted with debilitating scurvy because fresh fruits and vegetables were not storable aboard ship for long periods, and they lacked vitamin C when they went on long voyages.

Lind, on board the *Salisbury*, gathered sailors who were suffering from scurvy and divided them into several groups matched for severity and other factors. He then required that one group take 25 gutts of elixir vitriol daily, another group 2 spoonfuls of vinegar three times daily, another nutmeg, another oranges and lemons, while another group was allowed only a ration of seawater. Within days, dramatic change for the better occurred only in those eating the oranges and lemons.

Lind concluded that eating citrus fruits was essential to the diet of anyone who wished to avoid scurvy and that the disease was caused by the lack of these same fruits in the diet. The British Navy adopted the policy of serving its sailors limes and lime juice in 1795.

This experiment led Lind to the cause as well as to the treatment of scurvy, yet he did not choose to cause scurvy in the sailors by withholding citrus fruits from the sailors. They were already sick. In this instance, he felt no compunction about giving one group only seawater, which he regarded tantamount to no treatment, a strategy employed today usually with a group of sick people that constitutes a control group.

Ethical considerations can affect such decisions, and often such experiments avoid having a no-treatment group in favor of having several groups each treated differently but all treated with some accepted treatment. The groups are called comparison groups and provide data on which treatment of several possible ones is the best.

The data in *Cancer* present survival information collected from clinical treatment trials as researchers search for the most effective way to fight this disease. Some patients are given chemotherapy in different ways, some radiation treatments in different doses, others undergo surgery, and some receive all three when there is indication that these modalities in combination offer some success. As noted, survival for victims of a given kind of cancer can vary considerably, depending on the treatment.

Readers mindful of these many considerations and of the strategies used by medical researchers to determine what disease patterns exist and how they reveal possible causes of disease will better evaluate the information in this series. They will also better understand why controversy often rages within the medical community about the causes or treatment of disease. And they will better appreciate the remarkable progress achieved by epidemiologists, medical researchers, treating physicians, and policy makers in increasing average life expectancy and eliminating much pain and suffering from normal human existence.

Glossary

Age-adjusted rate: age adjustment, using the direct method, is the application of the age-specific death rates in a population of interest to a standardized age distribution to eliminate the differences in observed rates that result from differences in population composition.

Albuminuria: of albumin and serum protein in urine related to impaired renal function or strenuous exercise

Angiography: application of roentgen rays to examine blood vessels

Anorexia: loss of appetite

Antibody: a substance produced by the body that reacts with antigens

Antigen: a substance attacked by the body as foreign or harmful that unites with antibodies produced by the body during an immune reaction.

Azotemia: increased nitrogenous substances, such as urea, in the blood

Barium: an element that promotes sharp contrast imaging in X-ray films

Basal lamina: basement membrane

Cholangiogram: an X-ray film of the bile ducts

Cholesterol: a fat like substance in the blood, the brain, and all other tissues, cholesterol is manufactured by the liver and available through ingestion of animal products. It is necessary for the regulation of several body processes. Two forms include low-density lipoprotein (LDL) type and high density lipoprotein (HDL) type. A high level of circulating HDL is thought to prevent arteriosclerosis, while a high LDL reading is thought to contribute to heart disease

149

Cohort: any group of people with a common characteristic or set of characteristics studied or followed over time

Creatinine: the final product of creatine metabolism (methylglycyamidine $C_4H_7ON_3$), waste product from breakdown of creatine phosphate. Blood level of creatinine is an index of kidney function

Death rate: a measure that divides the number of deaths in a population in a given period by the resident population at the middle of that period

Dialysate: a water-concentrate solution used to absorb impurities in blood during dialysis of renal-failure patients

Discharge: according to the National Health Interview Survey the completion of any continuous period of stay of one or more nights in a hospital as an inpatient, excepting the stay of a well newborn infant

Duodenum: the first part of the small intestine

Dyspnea: difficulty in breathing

Endemic: characterizing a disease that occurs in a given locale on an ongoing basis

Endoscopy: a procedure involving insertion of a tubular optical device into an orifice or incision so that the inside of an organ or cavity can be inspected

Epithelial: referring to cells or tissues that line body cavities and the outer surface of the body

Febrile: feverish

Fistula: an abnormal opening

Flatulence: excess gas in the intestine or stomach

Focal: confined to a part of the whole

Gastritis: stomach inflammation

Gene: a segment of a chromosome containing a unit of genetic information and controlling a trait or process

Glucose: dextrose sugar

Hematocrit: proportion of erythrocytes in a volume of blood after centrifugation

Hematuria: blood in the urine

Hemoglobin: the pigment in red blood cells that contains oxygen

Histamine: produced from histadine at injury sites

Hormone: a substance made and secreted by a gland and carried by the bloodstream to other parts of the body, where it has a specific effect on body functions

Idiopathic: when the cause of disease cannot be determined

Incidence: the number of cases of disease having their onset during a particular interval, often expressed as a rate

Ischemic: obstructed blood flow

Life expectancy: the average years of life remaining to a person at a particular age based generally on the mortality conditions existing in the time mentioned

Malaise: discomfort or overall uneasiness accompanying infection

Mallory Weiss Syndrome: laceration of the distal esophagus and proximal stomach by vomiting, hiccups or drinking alcohol

Marital status: unmarried typically includes those who are single (never married), divorced or widowed, but the abortion surveillance reports of the Atlanta Centers for Disease Control count separated people as unmarried for all states except Rhode Island

Necrosis: dead area of tissues or bone

Nocturia: urination at night, interrupting sleep

Noninstitutionalized population: the population not residing in correctional institutions, detention homes, and training schools for delinquents, homes for the aged and dependent, homes for neglected children, the mentally or physically handicapped, unwed mothers, psychiatric or tuberculosis patients, and chronic disease hospitals. This population is the denominator in rates calculated for the National Center for Health Statistics' National Health Interview Survey, National Health and Nutrition Examination Survey, and National Ambulatory Medical Care Survey.

Oliguria: lessened urine formation

Palpable: detectable through touch

Peritoneum: the serous membrane lining of the abdominal cavity

Plasmapharesis: centrifuging blood to separate out red blood cells that can then be transferred instead of whole blood

Prevalence: the cases of a disease, number of infected persons, or of persons with some other attribute present during a particular interval; often expressed as a rate

Proteinuria: protein in the urine, usually as albumin

Pruritus: severe itching

Pyelonephritis: inflammation of the kidney due to infection

Pyuria: pus in the urine

Resident population: the population living in the United States including armed forces and resident foreigners excluding diplomats

Shunt: a device used to divert fluid flow, often blood, from one main route to another

Syndrome: a set of symptoms and signs occurring together

Ultrasound: a diagnostic technique in which pictures are made by bouncing sound waves off organs and other structures

Urea: substance formed in the liver from ammonia derived from amino acids

Varices: twisted veins

Xerophthalmia: conjunctival dryness following chronic conjunctivitis or vitamin-A deficiency

X-rays: high-energy radiation used in high doses to treat cancer or in low doses to diagnose the disease

Bibliography

Alter MJ, Gerety RJ, Smallwood LA, et al: Sporadic non-A, non-B hepatitis: frequency and epidemiology in an urban U.S. population. *J Infect Dis* 145:886–93, 1982

Armstrong JR, Daily RK, Dobson HL, et al: The incidence of glaucoma in diabetes mellitus. A comparison with the incidence of glaucoma in the general population. *Am J Ophthalmol* 50:55, 1960

Ashley A: Gamma globulin, effect on secondary attack rates in infectious hepatitis. *N Engl J Med* 250:412–417, 1954

Bachrach WH, Hofmann AF: Ursodeoxycholic acid in the treatment of cholesterol cholelithiasis. A review. *Dig Dis Sci* 23:737–761, 833–856, 1982

Basu TK: Impairment of absorption of ascorbic acid following ingestion of aspirin in guinea pigs. *Bioch Pharm* 31:4035–4038, 1982

Basu TK: Vitamin C-aspirin interactions. *Int J Vit Res* 23:83–90, 1982

Bell ET: A postmortem study of vascular disease in diabetics. *AMA Arch Pathol* 53:444, 1952

Bernier RH, Kane MA, Nalhanson N, et al: Issues related to the use of hepatitis B vaccine. *In* Millmon I (ed): Proceedings of the Symposium on Hepatitis B. The Virus, the Disease, and the Vaccine. Millmon I (ed): Philadelphia: Plenum Press, in press

Blumberg BS, et al: A serum antigen (Australia antigen) in Down's syndrome, leukemia and hepatitis. *Ann Intern Med* 66:924–931, 1967

Blumberg BS: Ira Hiscock lecture. Characteristics of the hepatitis B virus. *In* Genetic epidemiology, edited by New York, 1978, pp. 527–538

Blumberg BS, London WT: Hepatitis B virus and primary hepatocellular carcinoma: the relation of "Icrons" to cancer. *In* Viruses in naturally occurring cancers. Cold Spring Harbor Conference on Cell Proliferation, Sept. 4–9, 1979. Cold Spring Harbor Laboratory, Cold Spring Harbor, N.Y., vol 7, 1980, pp 401–421, in press.

Bonkalo AJ: Relation between Neuritis and the clinical background in diabetes mellitus. *Arch Intern Med* 85:944, 1950

Boyle D, Bhatia SK, Hadden DR, et al: Ischemic heart disease in diabetics. *Lancet* 1:338, 1972

Bradley RF, Bryfogle JW: Survival of diabetic patients after myocardial infarction. *Am J Med* 20:207, 1956

Brandman O, Redisch W: Incidence of peripheral vascular changes in diabetes mellitus: a survey of 264 cases. *Diabetes* 2:194, 1953

Brown LM, et al: Efficacy of vitamin supplementation in chronic alcoholics undergoing detoxification. *Alc Alcsm* 18:157–166, 1983

Bruyn GW, Garland H: Neuropathies of endocrine origin. *In* Vinken PJ, Bruyn GW (eds): Handbook of Neurology. Amsterdam: North Holland Publ. Co., 1970, vol 8, p 29

Burditt AF, Caird FI, Draper GJ: The natural history of diabetic retinopathy. *Q J Med* 37:303, 1968

Burditt AF, Caird FI: The natural history of lens opacities in diabetics. *Br J Ophthalmol* 52:433, 1968

Caird FI, Burditt AF, Draper GJ: Diabetic retinopathy. A further study of prognosis for vision. *Diabetes* 17:121, 1968

Caird FI: Survival of diabetics with proteinuria. *Diabetes* 10:178, 1961

Calne RY, Williams R, Lindop M, et al.: Improved survival after orthoptopic liver grafting. *Br Med J* 283:115, 1981

CDC. Hepatitis surveillance report No. 48, June 1982

CDC. Survey of viral hepatitis surveillance activities in state and local health departments. *MMWR* 30:164, 9–70, 1981

Colby AO: Neurologic disorders of diabetes mellitus, part I. *Diabetes* 14:516, 1965

Diabetes Mellitus. DHEW Publ. No. (NIH) 76-854, p 1, 1976

Elson CO, Graeff AS, James SP, et al: Covert suppressor T cells in Crohn's disease. *Gastroenterology* 80:1513, 1981

Epstein FH, Ostrander, LD, Johnson BC, et al: Epidemiological studies of cardiovascular disease in a total community—Tecumseh, Michigan. *Ann Intern Med* 62:1170, 1965

Etzwiler DD: Incidence of urinary-tract infections among juvenile diabetics. JAMA 191:93 1965

Francis DP, Hadler SC, Thompson SE, et al: The prevention of hepatitis B with vaccine. Report of the Centers for Disease Control multi-center efficacy trial among homosexual men. *Ann Intern Med* 97:362–366, 1982

Francis DP, Maynard JE. The transmission and outcome of hepatitis A, B, and non-A, non-B: review. *Epidemiol Rev* 1:17–31 1979

Fraser DM, Campbell IW, Ewing DJ, et al: Peripheral and autonomic nerve function in newly diagnosed diabetes mellitus. *Diabetes* 26:546, 1977

Garcia MJ, McNamara PM, Gordon, T, et al: Morbidity and mortality in diabetics in the Framingham population. *Diabetes* 23:105, 1974

Glover J: Factors affecting vitamin A transport in animals and man. *Proc Nutr Soc* 42:95–101, 1983

Goldner MG: The fate of the second leg in the diabetic amputee. *Diabetes* 9:100, 1960

Hadler SC, Erben JJ, Francis DP, et al: Risk factors for hepatitis A in day-care centers. *J Infect Dis* 145:255–61, 1982

Hadler SC, Erben JJ, Matthews D, et al: Effect of immunoglobulin on hepatitis A in day-care centers. *JAMA* 249:48–53, 1983

Hofmann AF: Gallstone-dissolving drugs. New approach to an old disease. *Drug Therapy* 12:57–71, 1982

Hofmann AF: The medical treatment of cholesterol gallstones: a major advance in preventive gastroenterology (editorial). *Am J Med* 69:4–7, 1980

Knowles HC, Jr: Long-term juvenile diabetes treated with unmeasured diet. *Trans Assoc Am Phys* 84:95, 1971

Knowles HC, Jr: Magnitude of the renal failure problem in diabetic patients. *Kidney International* 6, (4), Suppl 1: New York: Springer-Verlag, 1974

Knowles HC, Jr, Guest GM, Lampe J, et al: The course of juvenile diabetes treated with unmeasured diet. *Diabetes* 14:239, 1965

Kramer DW, Perilstein PK: Peripheral vascular complications in diabetes mellitus. A survey of 3,600 cases. *Diabetes* 7:384, 1958

Liebow IM, Hellerstein HK, Miller M: Arteriosclerotic heart disease in diabetes mellitus: a clinical study of 383 patients. *Am J Med* 18:438, 1955

London WT, Sutnick AI, Blumberg BS: Australia antigen and acute viral hepatitis. *Ann Intern Med* 70:55–59 (1969)

Massry, SG: Parathyroid Hormone and Uremia 5 ROI AM 29955-01. Los Angeles: University of Southern California

Maynard JE: Hepatitis B vaccine: strategies for utilization. *In* Maupas P, Guesry P (eds): Hepatitis B Vaccine Inserm, Symposium No. 18. Amsterdam: Elsevier North Holland Biomedical Press. 1981, pp 13–19

National Center for Health Statistics: Comparison of hospitalization reporting in three survey procedures. *Vital and Health Statistics.* PHS Pub. No. 1000-Series 2-No. 8. Public Health Service. Washington. U.S. Government Printing Office, July 1965

National Center for Health Statistics: Estimation and sampling variance in the Health Interview Survey. *Vital and Health Statistics.* PHS Pub. No. 1000-Series 2-No. 38. Public Health Service. Washington. U.S. Government Printing Office, June 1970

National Center for Health Statistics: Health interview responses compared with medical records. *Vital and Health Statistics.* PHS Pub. No. 1000-Series 2-No. 7. Public Health Service. Washington. U.S. Government Printing Office. July 1965

National Center for Health Statistics: Health Interview Survey procedure, 1957–1974. *Vital and Health Statistics.* Series 1-No. 11. DHEW Pub. No. (HRA) 75-1311. Health Resources Administration. Washington. U.S. Government Printing Office, April 1975

National Center for Health Statistics: Health survey procedure: concepts, questionnaire development, and definitions in the Health Interview Survey, *Vital and Health Statistics.* PHS Pub. No. 1000-Series 1-No. 2. Public Health Service. Washington. U.S. Government Printing Office, May 1964

National Center for Health Statistics: Interview data on chronic conditions compared with information derived from medical records. *Vital and Health Statistics.* PHS Pub. No. 1000-Series 2-No. 23. Public Health Service. Washington. U.S. Government Printing Office, May 1967

National Center for Health Statistics: Quality control and measurement of nonsampling error in the Health Interview Survey. *Vital and Health Statistics.* Series 2-No. 54. DHEW Pub. No. (HSM) 73-1328. Health Services and Mental Health Administration. Washington. U.S. Government Printing Office, Mar. 1973

Opelz G, Sengar DPS, et al: Effect of blood transfusions on subsequent kidney transplants. *Transplant Proc* 5:253, 1973

Opelz G, Terasaki PI: Importance of preoperative transfusions for cadaver kidney transplants. *Transplantation* 31:106, 1981

Partamian JO, Bradley RF: Acute myocardial infarction in 258 cases of diabetes. Immediate mortality and five-year survival. *New Engl J Med* 273:455, 1965

Patz A, Berkow JW: Visual and systemic prognosis in diabetic retinopathy. *Trans Am Acad Ophthalmol Otolaryngol* 72:253, 1968

Pell S, D'Alonzo A: Some aspects of hypertension in diabetes mellitus. *JAMA* 202:104, 1967

Proceedings of the NIH consensus workshop on upper gastrointestinal bleed.   Dis. Dig. Sci. 26:1S–102S, 1981

Public Health Service Advisory Committee on Immunization Practices: Immune globulins for protection against viral hepatitis. *MMWR* 26:425–428, 1977

Report of the National Commission on Diabetes.   DHEW Publ. No. (NIH) 76–1022, vol 3, pt 2, p 35, 1975

Richardson GG, Cook DA: Effect of dietary fat on B-carotene bioavailability. *Fed Proc* 42:811, 1983

Robert A: Cytoprotection by prostaglandins. *Gastroenterology* 77:761–767, 1979

Robert A: Prostaglandins and the digestive tract. In Johnson LR (ed): Physiology of the Gastrointestinal Tract. New York: Raven Press, 1981, pp 1407–1434

Root HF, Mirsky S, Ditzel J: Proliferative retinopathy in diabetes mellitus. Review of eight hundred forty-seven cases. *JAMA* 169:903, 1959

Schreeder MT, Thompson SE, Hadler SC, et al: Hepatitis B in homosexual men: prevalence of infection and factors related to transmission. *J Infect Dis* 146:7–15 1982

Sharpey-Schafer EP, Taylor PB: Absent circulatory reflexes in diabetic neuritis. *Lancet* 1:559, 1960

Smith JA, O'Connor JJ, Willis AT: Nasal carriage of *Staphylococcus aureus* in diabetes mellitus. *Lancet* 2:776, 1966

Smolle J, Wawschin O, Hayn H, et al: (GE) Serum levels of vitamin A and carotene in thyroid-disease. *Acta Med Aust*, 10:71–73, 1983

Starzl TE, Iwatuski S, Van Thiel DH, *et al*:   Evolution of liver transplantation. *Hepatology*, 2:614, 1982

Starzl TE, Putman CW, Hansbrough JF, *et al*:   Biliary complications after liver transplantation; with special reference to the biliary cast syndrome and techniques of secondary duct repair. *Surgery* 81:212, 1977

Szmuness W, et al: Sociodemographic aspects of the epidemiology of hepatitis B. Vyas GN, Cohen SN, Schmid R (eds): *Viral Hepatitis.* Philadelphia: Franklin Institute Press, 1978, pp 297–320

Szmuness W, Stevens CE, Harley EJ, et al: Hepatitis B vaccine. Demonstration of efficacy in a controlled clinical trial in a high risk population in the United States. *N Engl J Med* 303:833–841, Oct 9, 1980

Thistle, JL, Carlson, GL, Hofmann, AF, LaRusso NF, MacCarty RL, Flynn GL, Higuchi WI, and Babayan VK. Mono-octanoin, a Dissolution Agent for Retained Cholesterol Bile Duct Stones: Physical Properties and Clinical Application. *Gastroenterology* 78:1016–1022, 1980

Tolsma DD, Bryan JA: The economic impact of viral hepatitis in the United States. Public Health Rep 91:349–353, 1976

Tuazon C, Perez A, Kishaba T, Sheagren JN: Staphylococcus Aureus Among Insulin-Injecting Diabetic Patients. *JAMA* 231:1272, 1975

Klimt CR, Knatterud GL, Meinert CL, et al: A study of the effects of hypoglycemic agents on vascular complications in patients with adult-onset diabetes. Part I. Design, methods and baseline characteristics. *Diabetes* 19(suppl 2):747, 1970

U.S. National Health Survey: The statistical design of the health household interview survey. *Health Statistics.* PHS Pub. No. 584-A2. Public Health Service. Washington. D.C., July 1958

Walsh JH: Gastrointestinal hormones and peptides. *In* Johnson LR (ed): Physiology of the Gastrointestinal Tract. New York: Raven Press, 1981, pp. 57–145

Ward JD, Barnes CG, Fisher DJ, et al: Improvement in nerve conduction following treatment in newly diagnosed diabetics. *Lancet* 1:428, 1971

Way LW: The National Cooperative Gallstone Study and chenodiol. *Gastroenterology* 84:648–651, 1983

White P: Natural course and prognosis of juvenile diabetes. *Diabetes* 5:445, 1956

Whitehouse FW: Infections that hospitalize the diabetic. *Geriatrics* 28:97, 1973

Whitehouse FW, Jurgensen C, Block M: The later life of the diabetic amputee. Another look at the fate of the second leg. *Diabetes* 17:520, 1968

INDEX